The Baby Bible

The Baby Bible
Choosing the Best for You and Your Baby

Juliet Leigh

VICTOR GOLLANCZ
LONDON

First published as a Gollancz Paperback Original 1996
by Victor Gollancz
An imprint of the Cassell Group
Wellington House, 125 Strand, London WC2R 0BB

© Juliet Leigh 1996

All rights reserved. No part of this publication may be reproduced or transmitted in any form or by any means, electronic or mechanical including photocopying, recording or any information storage or retrieval system, without prior permission in writing from the publishers.

The right of Juliet Leigh to be identified as author of this work has been asserted by her in accordance with the Copyright, Designs and Patents Act, 1988.

Illustrations by Viv Quillin

A catalogue record for this book is available from the British Library.

ISBN 0 575 06034 4

Photoset in Great Britain by
Rowland Phototypesetting Ltd, Bury St Edmunds, Suffolk
Printed and bound in Guernsey by
The Guernsey Press Co. Ltd, Guernsey, Channel Islands

96 97 98 99   10 9 8 7 6 5 4 3 2 1

*This book is for all my family but especially
Trevor, Tom and Annabel*

Contents

Acknowledgements	11
Introduction	13

PART ONE: PREGNANCY

1: Healthcare Options — 17
- Choosing a Hospital — 18
- Choices in Care — 20
- Tests and Screening — 30
- Genetic Counselling — 37
- Antenatal Classes — 38
- Multiple Pregnancy — 42
- Disability and Pregnancy — 45

2: Taking Care of Yourself — 48
- Your Diet — 48
- Medicines and Pregnancy — 53
- Beauty During Pregnancy — 54
- Maternity Bras — 59
- Maternity Clothes — 62
- Travelling When Pregnant — 66

3: Law and Finance — 68
- Pregnant Women at Work — 68
- Benefits — 72
- Financial Planning for You and Your New Baby — 76

PART TWO: PARENTS AS CONSUMERS

4: Buying and Hiring — 89
- Shopping for Your Baby — 89
- Equipment Hire — 100
- British Standards — 102

5: Safety — 105
- Avoiding Accidents — 105
- Babies and Other Animals — 114

6: The Green Parent — 117
- Pregnancy and the Environment — 117
- Complementary Medicines and Therapies — 120
- Your Baby and the Environment — 128

PART THREE: GIVING BIRTH

7: The Big Day — 137
- Birth Plans — 137
- Choices for Pain Relief — 139
- What to Pack for Hospital — 145
- Premature Babies — 147
- Toiletries for Postnatal Mothers — 150

8: Registration and Celebration — 152
- Registering Your Baby's Birth — 152
- Choosing Your Baby's Name — 153
- Ceremonies to Mark the Birth — 155
- Buying a Gift for a New Baby — 160

9: Parents and Carers — 164
- Fatherhood — 164
- Single Parenthood — 167
- Childcare — 169

PART FOUR: GETTING TO THE BOTTOM OF IT

10: Changing Your Baby — 187
- Nappies — 187
- Nappy Changes — 192

PART FIVE: BATHTIME
11: In the Bathroom — 199
- Baby Baths — 199
- Baby Toiletries — 201
- The Bathroom Cabinet — 203

PART SIX: THE NURSERY
12: Preparing the Nursery — 207
- Decorating a Nursery — 207
- Nursery Furniture — 213

13: Bedtime — 218
- Cots and Cotbeds — 218
- Moses Baskets — 226
- Comforters and Soothers — 228
- Baby Monitors — 230

PART SEVEN: EATING
14: Feeding Your Baby — 235
- Breasts and Breastfeeding — 235
- Bottle Feeding — 243
- Baby Foods — 253
- Highchairs and Baby Diners — 258

PART EIGHT: GETTING AROUND
15: Baby Transport — 265
- Slings — 265
- Car Seats — 266
- Prams and Buggies — 274
- Cycling with a Baby — 287

16: Travel — 291

PART NINE: FASHION, FUN AND GAMES
17: Dressing — 299
- Baby Clothes — 299
- Washing Baby Clothes — 303

18: Playtime   305
  Toys   305
  Playpens   313
  Bouncy Chairs   314

PART TEN: COPING
19: Dealing with Problems   317
  The Pressure Pregnancy Places on Relationships   317
  Losing Your Baby Through Miscarriage or Stillbirth   317
  Conceiving Again   321
  Adoption and Fostering   325
  When Things Go Wrong with the Birth   326
  'Baby Blues' and Postnatal Depression   332
  Sleep Problems   335

Appendices
  Pregnancy Checklist   337
  The Essentials   340
  Further Reading   343

Index   345

Acknowledgements

The Baby Bible would not have been born without help from the following: Angela Brand, Trevor Leigh, Andrew Lownie, the team at Gollancz, especially Vicki Harris, Katrina Whone and Liz Knights; also Morris and Manja Leigh, and John Harris, James and Josephine Chambers, Katy and Paul Templeton. Krystyna Grant, who did a mammoth job in a minute time, co-ordinating the research – I am grateful to you all.

Many health professionals gave up valuable time to help. Their experience and expertise was greatly appreciated. In particular, Mr Frank Loeffler, Dr Janet Cresswell, Dr Tony Blackett and Charlotte Young at Sheffield; Dr Peter Mason, Dr Simon Moore, Dr Helen Murphy, Susan Tanner, Dr Gill Harris, Dr Walter Barker, Lyn Carlton, Andrew Dawood, Cathy McCormick of the Royal College of Midwives; and Ann Graveley of *Midwife* magazine. The Kent team of midwives at the Chelsea and Westminster Hospital, the health visitors of Walmer Road Health Clinic, London; Trish Muncaster and Beryl Bennington and new mothers of the Gayton Road Health Centre, King's Lynn; Pat Young and expectant parents and new mothers at the Horsforth Health Clinic, Leeds; and Anita O'Neil, St John and St Elizabeth Birth Unit, London, Tony Ashwell, Dial UK. The wonderful women of Parentability, especially Ruth Carter and Clare Burnell of Choices in Childcare.

The National Childbirth Trust postnatal co-ordinators have been phenomenal in their assistance and enthusiasm. Nicola Clarke of Cuidu/Irish Childbirth Trust was phenomenally kind and efficient. I would particularly like to thank those many new mothers who crawled out of their homes after sleepless nights with their new babies to attend discussion groups on 'best buys'; also NCT Postnatal co-ordinators Kathleen Pajak, Stirling; Clare Eadie, Edinburgh East; Angela Hind, West Clwyd; Catherine

Roper, Glasgow South; Fiona Bradley, Blackpool; Veronica Dunne, Lancaster; Lucy Clark and Genevieve Kilby, Guildford; Caroline Wright, Cambridge; Margaret Jones, Loughborough; Sally Spencer, Hull; Priscilla White, Plymouth; Caroline Avey, Epping; Katherine New, Teignmouth; Caroline Sidebottom, Peterborough; Janet Cartwright, Leeds; Beverley Walters, Sandra Kitching, Birmingham; Deborah Digby, Cheshire; Deborah Pennycock, Perth; Michelle Broughton, Wirral; Joanna Rufus, Dorchester; Lisa Goldsmith, North Cornwall; Hilary Graves, Crawley; Mandy Gannon, Basingstoke; Nikki Macfarlane, Bishop's Cleeve. The following 'star' NNEBs enlightened me on the question of best buys and were enthusiastic product testers: Kate Lees, Belinda North, Alison Knight; Fiona Hockenhull, Head of Teddies Nursery, Fulham, London, and her staff – in particular Elise Beaumont, Celia Treneer-Michell, Bronwen Stainsby and Claire Adams. Also Juliet Pick, Susan Leighton, Howard Leigh, Tim Kahn, Parent Network, countless staff at Boots the Chemist, Sarah Entwistle of Baby Equipment Hire and Alison Walters of the Nursery Hire Shop; Douglas Simmons, Carol Ross, Sylvia Baker, AOC; Aysha Malik at the Office of Population and Census Surveys; Suzanne Strong; Sandra Levinson; Dawn Jones, President of Central London Twins Club; Gina Siddons, TAMBA co-ordinator.

Robert Chantry-Price, Secretary of The Baby Products Association, was unstintingly generous with time and information. As were librarians Patricia Donnithorne and Eileen Abbott at the National Childbirth Trust headquarters.

Last but perhaps most importantly, I owe a huge debt to my own gruesome twosome who unwittingly tested a vast variety of products. I pray that these experiences have left them less psychologically damaged than their mother.

I have tried as far as possible to approach all organizations mentioned in the book regarding their entry, but I may inadvertently have missed some. I apologize in advance for any omissions.

Introduction

Our first pram was meant to be a luxury, 'easy-fold' model, and for a trained engineer it probably was. Six months later the frame was twisted out of recognition and the pram met a sudden, well-deserved end when my husband threw it down the front steps.

Three years later I ventured into the pram market again. I had learned from my mistakes and bought a model that was cheap and cheerful. The pram was cheap. I was miserable. This zappy little thing had wandering wheel problems. It perpetually veered towards the kerb, dragging myself, the baby and screeching toddler in a drunken fashion through the streets of West London.

I won't bore you with the sagas of what happened when the buggy met the washing machine, with the collapse of the cot or with the countless accidents caused by a particular 'safety' device. But I was beginning to see that I had an unerring nose for buying duds. Then I started talking to my friends.

I realized that most parents have had similar experiences, and found it hard to admit that they have ever bought a useless piece of kit, which might reflect on them as 'bad' parents, out of touch with the needs of their babies. But nearly everyone has made a purchase that they have come to regret.

More importantly, those who experienced problems during pregnancy or early parenthood were irritated when they later discovered a particular organization or product that could have helped them, if only they had known at the time. What was needed was a comprehensive guide. The seeds of *The Baby Bible* were sown.

The Baby Bible was initially designed to answer all the questions I needed answers for when I was pregnant. It rapidly expanded as hundreds of people – mothers, medical experts, retailers, manufacturers and voluntary organizations – helped by suggesting services and items they found useful. Despite the diversity of people canvased, there was a surprising amount of agreement over which brands really stood the test of time and which services were especially helpful.

Most people want to spoil a new baby but everyone has a different outlook on how to go about it. No one likes to feel they have been 'done'. This book is designed to help families make choices that will suit them – whatever their needs, taste or budget.

Babies are referred to as either 'he' or 'she' throughout to avoid the laborious 'he or she'.

The information included in *The Baby Bible* is as accurate as we could make it at the time of going to press. Details of price and availability will undoubtedly date quickly, and we apologize for any inaccuracies. The omission of any particular brand, company or any other organization implies neither censure nor recommendation. As a general rule, when buying through mail order it is advisable to telephone first.

Help us to make the Baby Bible better
If you have found any excellent products or services that are not mentioned in *The Baby Bible*, please get in touch to let us know. Information should go to Mr D. Reed, Baby Bible, 172 Greenford Road, Harrow, Middlesex HA1 3QZ.

Juliet Leigh

PART ONE
PREGNANCY

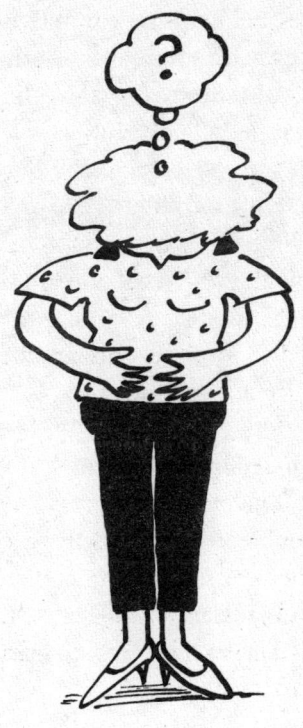

1   Healthcare Options

If you are not already pregnant, please turn to Chapter 19 for information on pregnancy and ovulation tests, and fertility problems.

The last few years have seen the publication of two government reports which have had a dramatic effect on Britain's maternity services. It is now officially recognized that pregnant women should be allowed to express a preference where they have their babies – at home or in hospital – and who will be chiefly responsible for their antenatal care. This can be a doctor, a midwife or a combination of professionals. Always remember that your carer or carers may fall ill or be on holiday when your baby arrives, so continuity of care can never be guaranteed.

The Citizen's Charter and childbirth

In 1994, the government launched the 'New Maternity Charter'. The key rights and standards are:
- You have the right to choose where your baby is born – in hospital or at home.
- You can choose who will be with you – husband, partner, friend or relative – during labour and birth.
- You should be told the name of the midwife who will be responsible for your midwifery care.
- You have the right to see your records during pregnancy and, if you choose, to keep them with you rather than leave them with the hospital, GP or midwife.

- You should be given a specific time for appointments and seen within thirty minutes of that time.
- Your local Community Health Council can also provide help and advice. Their contact details will be listed under 'Community Health Council' in the telephone directory.
- If you have concerns about the service you are receiving, in the first instance tell the people involved – your doctor or postnatal clinic. If that does not work, contact the Health Information Service on 0800 665544. They should be able to help. They also provide a booklet entitled 'The Patient's Charter on Maternity Services'.
- AIMS – The Association for Improvements in the Maternity Services, tel: 0181 960 5585 – is a good source of advice and support for women who are unhappy with their maternity care (address on page 21). AIMS are also in Ireland. Tel: 280 4161/286 4585.

Choosing a Hospital

You often have little time to make the crucial decision on where to give birth. Popular hospitals get booked up early. On talking to friends and health professionals, you may find that one local hospital is 'flavour of the month', but it is still worth finding out about the alternatives. You may have a choice between teaching hospitals and community hospitals. Teaching hospitals train medical professionals, and even if the buildings themselves seem on the point of collapse, they should have extensive modern facilities. Community hospitals tend to be smaller and more personal, but they may not have the same level of technology as teaching hospitals.

Some areas have GP units, which are either part of a hospital or exist on their own, where your GP can supervise the delivery of your baby. A midwife will probably be responsible for the delivery itself, but your GP will follow up with your postnatal care. If there are complications during the birth, you may need to be transferred to a more sophisticated labour ward.

Find Out From Your GP

Find out from your GP or the hospitals themselves whether you can see the facilities. Some hospitals have regular tours. Alternatively, the hospital might arrange for you to be shown round on your own. If the hospital you like is inconvenient for your home, find out from your GP if a shared-care/Domino option is possible (see page 22).

Before you go on your visit, prepare your questions in advance. You should consider the following points:

Questions to ask

- Does the hospital run antenatal classes?
- What subjects are covered?
- What time are they held?
- Are there classes for partners?
- Will I be able to build up relationships with a group of midwives, so that there is a good chance I will know the midwife who is present at the birth?
- Is one of the group available on the phone twenty-four hours a day?
- Will the midwives make a point of sitting down and working out a birth plan with me?
- Am I allowed to move around and find a position I feel comfortable with to give birth?
- Does the same midwife stay with me throughout labour?
- Do they have a 'home-from-home' birthing suite for low-risk births? (see information on Royal Victoria Infirmary and Leeds General Infirmary on pages 24–5).
- Are water births common? If not, is it possible to labour in water or to bring in a birthing pool?
- Is there a special-care baby unit? If not, what happens if the baby is sick?

- How long is the average hospital stay?
- What sort of accommodation will I be given?
- Do midwives actively promote breastfeeding? If so, how?
- Can my partner stay at the hospital?
- Can family and friends visit at any time?
- Does the baby stay with me all the time, or is there a nursery?
- Is the maternity unit secure? How are the babies kept safe from strangers?
- Does the hospital run any postnatal exercise classes or postnatal groups?

Once you have decided which hospital is for you, you need to decide how much of your antenatal care takes place there; it can be all of it, or just the birth and certain tests.

Choices in Care

The National Health Service

The following pages offer a brief run-down of the choices available, but there are differences between one area and the next, and you are strongly advised to talk to your GP and other local mothers before making a decision.

If you are the first of your family or friends to be having a baby in the area, your local National Childbirth Trust (NCT) branch will be able to advise you or put you in touch with women who have recently had babies at nearby hospitals. Telephone their head office on 0181 992 8637 for the number of your closest co-ordinator.

There are also numerous excellent books on pregnancy and birth (see the lists at the back of the book).

If you do not want to go to your own GP you can either:
- choose another by contacting your local Family Practitioners Committee (this will be listed in your phone book); or

- go to another GP just for your maternity care even if you wish to stay with your usual GP for any other problems.

If you are a few months into your pregnancy and are unhappy with the care you are receiving and you would like expert advice, contact **AIMS**, the Association for Improvement in the Maternity Services, 40 Kingswood Avenue, London NW6 6LS, tel. 0181 960 5585. AIMS also houses Vaginal Birth After Caesarean (**VBAC**). If you want advice before or after a Caesarean delivery, call NCT head office 0181 992 8637 and ask to be put in touch with a Caesarean Birth/VBAC co-ordinator. Say whether you want antenatal or postnatal advice as there are particular co-ordinators for both. People living in Eire could contact the Caesarean Support Group (Eire) 295 4953.

Consultant/Hospital Care

If you choose this option, appointments all take place in the hospital, where you will usually see a consultant obstetrician or one of his/her team. However, there are exceptions to this rule. In many units, care is provided by an integrated team of doctors and midwives of which the consultant is a member.

PLUS POINTS
* There are resources to spot and deal with medical conditions and complications immediately.
* In some hospitals there is a strong emphasis on continuity of care, so you will have months to build up a rapport with the midwives who will support you during labour and after the birth.
* The hospital environment becomes familiar.

MINUS POINTS
* You may never meet the consultant and you cannot be sure who will be with you during labour if you are seen by a different doctor or midwife at each appointment.
* Travelling to the hospital and waiting to be seen can take a long time.

Shared Care

Shared care means that your antenatal care is shared between your GP's surgery and the hospital. Apart from your scan and any specialist tests carried out in the hospital, you see either your GP at the local surgery or a community midwife.

PLUS POINTS
* Continuity of care. You can build up a close relationship with a small team of midwives.
* This option is well suited to arranging a home birth.
* It may be more convenient to go to your GP rather than to the hospital for routine appointments.
* Your GP knows your medical history.

MINUS POINT
* If you give birth in hospital, you are unlikely to have met the midwife who cares for you in labour.

The Domino Scheme

This is very similar to shared care. Your antenatal care is divided between your GP and a local team of community midwives. Your community midwife usually delivers your baby. You go into hospital for the birth and leave within six to twenty-four hours afterwards.

PLUS POINTS
* Continuity of care. Two of the midwives whom you already know will deliver your baby.
* You can leave hospital quickly after the birth.

MINUS POINT
* If you have problems following the birth you will have to go back into hospital, even though you have already been discharged.

Midwife-led Care

The supervisor at your local maternity unit may be able to book you into the unit for antenatal and postnatal care and tell them if you are considering a home birth. In some areas you may have to go through your GP.

You are seen by midwives, either in your home or at your local clinic. You will get to know the whole team of midwives, one of whom will be there for your delivery.

> **PLUS POINTS**
> * Continuity of care.
> * A familiar face will be there at the birth, whether it is at home or in hospital.
>
> **MINUS POINT**
> * This scheme is only suitable for low-risk women. If a complication arises, you may have to change to hospital-led care.

A Small Taste of What the NHS Can Offer

The **Christiana Hartley Maternity Hospital, Southport**, can offer the ultimate experience in relaxation therapy to mothers before, during and after labour: the 'Sensations Suite' or Snoezelen Room. This consists of thick wall-to-wall cushioning and beanbags, which women can move and mould for their comfort. There are bubble tubes; star panels of multicoloured lights; wind-chimes; a projector reflecting rotating patterns of light on to the white walls; an aromatherapy atomizer and a cassette deck with a choice of soothing relaxation tapes. By pressing a series of switches the woman can decide which facility to operate.

The **All Saints Hospital (Medway NHS Trust) Chatham, Kent**, has an unusual range of services. Your midwife can arrange foetal monitoring at home, with data being sent via the telephone and analysed on a computer screen back at the hospital. Eight per cent of their births take place at home, a higher percentage than the national average. They have a group of midwives trained in signing for deaf mothers and deaf partners and a minicom on the labour ward for their use. Midwives are also trained in baby massage, which they teach to new mothers.

The **Royal Victoria Infirmary, Newcastle-upon-Tyne**, has a midwifery-led unit for low-risk births. Staff do not wear uniform, and there is a home-from-home atmosphere with fitted carpets and attractive decoration. There are double beds to enable partners to stay and any equipment is hidden away in cupboards and drawers. Medical intervention is not available in the birthing room, but if you do decide you need an epidural, you simply go through the swing doors into the central maternity unit. The RVI believes that continuity of care is of paramount importance, and advice and support is given to mothers for up to sixteen weeks following the birth.

Not far away, at the **South Tyneside District Hospital**, tremendous efforts have been made to ensure the best possible service for the community. An advice centre is planned for the South Shields branch of Mothercare and expectant and new mothers are encouraged to drop in to the maternity unit with any questions they might have. Parents of special-care babies have the advantage of knowing that a community-link midwife will visit all babies discharged from the special-care baby unit for as long as the family requires their help and support.

The **Aberdeen Royal Hospital NHS Trust** can also offer a midwifery-led unit which is very receptive to special requests. For example, mothers can bring in pools for water births if they want to. At the **Perth Royal Infirmary** there is a particularly well-run antenatal class where a midwife and fitness instructor hold exercising-to-music sessions for expectant mothers as well as discussing the medical aspects of pregnancy with them.

The **Leeds General Infirmary** has a 'home-from-home' suite which includes a sitting/dining room and a jacuzzi. Mothers report how relaxed they felt going into this environment to have their babies. Some of the midwives are trained aromatherapists.

In Wales, the **Taff Ely Rhondda Midwifery Service** aims to deliver a women-centred approach to care. Sixty-five per cent of women are cared for by Know Your Midwife teams who are community based and work closely with local GPs. The midwives offer aquanatal classes and individualized preparation-for-parenthood programmes in community settings.

Wales seems particularly strong on offering a caring service to expectant mothers. The **Llandough Hospital and Community NHS Trust** comes highly recommended for its integrated midwifery system, which gives expectant mothers twenty-four-hour access to a midwife, usually one she knows. After the birth, postnatal visits continue according to individual needs.

The **St Helier NHS Trust, Carshalton, Surrey**, offers not only water births but also community midwives who provide massage. Zita West at **Warwick Hospital** is a midwife acupuncturist who can offer treatment on the NHS for conditions related to pregnancy and postnatal health, e.g., morning sickness, backache, sciatica and carpal tunnel syndrome. **Derriford Maternity Unit, Plymouth**, also boasts midwife acupuncturists.

At the **Royal Devon and Exeter Hospital**, also known as the **Heavitree**, massage is available to pregnant women and new mothers from two qualified midwife masseuses. They also teach massage skills as part of their parentcraft programme. In addition there is a full-time counsellor for expectant mothers who feel stressed or worried. **Derby City General Hospital** can offer aquanatal classes, aromatherapy from a qualified midwife aromatherapist, hypnotherapy and a signing midwife for deaf women. The hospital also has a specialist baby-feeding adviser.

For those particularly anxious to breastfeed, at the **Queen's**

Medical Centre, Nottingham, there is an expert on breast-feeding to help mothers individually. Interpreters for Asian language speakers are also employed and a staffed play area is provided in the antenatal clinic. Water births are encouraged and a plumbed-in birthing pool is available.

The **Liverpool Maternity Hospital** has a 'Back to the Future' team of midwives who have devised a model of care specifically to suit the needs of the women of Liverpool. Women who are allocated to the team meet all the team members during the course of their pregnancy and are usually delivered by someone they know.

St Mary's Hospital, Paddington in London, is a large teaching hospital which provides mothers with a high level of personal attention as well as first-class facilities. Water births and midwife-only care schemes are available as well as a superb special-care baby unit. Mobile epidurals are now offered so that labouring mothers can be given this type of pain relief without having to be confined to bed.

At the other end of the spectrum is the **Grantham and District Hospital NHS Trust**, where 'small is beautiful' – as they put it themselves, they are 'large enough to cater, but small enough to care'. Mothers living outside Grantham can attend antenatal clinics nearer home and labours in water can be arranged. The **Cheviot and Wansbeck NHS Trust** in Northumberland also offers close personal contact, through its two small GP/midwife units at Berwick and Alnwick. There is special expertise in water births at Ashington Maternity Unit.

The **Leicester Royal Infirmary NHS Trust** has offered a 'home from home' unit since 1988. This has six delivery rooms, furnished to resemble normal bedrooms, in which women are encouraged to play an active role in their own labour. The unit has its own kitchen and bathroom, and welcomes partners. Water-birth facilities are available. Postnatal care is enhanced by the Breastfeeding Helpline.

If you live in the Winchester area and are concerned about

having a baby following a previous bad experience, the **Royal Hampshire Maternity Hospital** (answerphone 01962 824606) has started 'Birth Afterthoughts', a service for women who have unanswered questions that can trouble them for months or, in one case, up to twenty-two years after a birth. Parents can meet a midwife, ask questions about the birth and see their maternity notes. These discussions often help partners to deal with any feelings of guilt or blame and influences the hospital in its own practice and attitudes.

Having Your Baby at Home

PLUS POINTS
* You may feel more comfortable in familiar surroundings.
* Your midwife will stay with you until the baby is born.
* Your partner can feel more involved.

MINUS POINTS
* This option is only suitable for low-risk mothers.
* Your GP may be against it, so you might have to change doctors to have a home birth.
* It is harder to monitor the health of the baby.
* If anything goes wrong with you or your baby, you will have to rush to hospital.
* You may be desperate for more pain relief than can be offered at home.
* The house will have to be organized and then cleaned up.

For information on and support in choosing a home birth, contact the **International Home Birth Movement**, Standlake Manor, Witney, Oxfordshire OX8 7RH, tel. 01865 300154. **The Home Birth Centre** in Eire (tel. 492 2565) will advise Irish women. The **NCT** (National Childbirth Trust) (tel. 0181 992 8637) will be able to put you in touch with a local support group.

Private Medicine

Independent Midwives

Independent midwives work outside the NHS. You employ them privately to do all your antenatal checks and deliver your baby either at home or in a private or NHS hospital. There are not too many around, so telephone the Independent Midwives Association on 0181 406 3172 to find out what services are available in your area.

> **PLUS POINTS**
> * As midwives usually work in pairs, you will be able to build up a strong relationship with them.
> * If you are anxious to have a birth where you feel in control, independent midwives make excellent facilitators as they are employed by you and do not have to fit in with hospital policies – except in an emergency, of course.
>
> **MINUS POINT**
> * Cost. Between £900 and £2,800.

There are two major centres of expertise for private midwifery. The **Wessex Maternity Centre**, Mansbridge Road, West End, Southampton, Hants SO18 3HW, tel. 01703 464721, an independent maternity centre offering a full range of services from antenatal classes through to home births. There is a suite designed to cater for wheelchair-bound women or their partners. Although you do not have to be giving birth at the centre to enjoy their classes, there is a good chance that many of their services will be available on the NHS at some point during 1996. For a full care package, including antenatal care and a birth at the centre, expect to pay £900 for a first baby and £700 for subsequent births.

The **Special Delivery Midwifery Practice Centre**, 34 Elm Quay Court, Nine Elms Lane, London SW8 5DE, tel. 0171 498 2322, is run by two highly respected midwives, Caroline Flint and Valerie Taylor, who believe in 'giving birth back to the mother'. They offer full antenatal care and cater for home births as well as supplying various facilities, including a birthing pool in each room in their own birth centre. This is adjacent to a major London teaching hospital, so women can be admitted to a high-tech maternity unit within minutes if necessary. Their package starts at around £2,450 and goes up to £2,750 for a birth in the centre. The practice can also arrange for a private-hospital birth, a Japanese-speaking midwife and a mother's help package: eighty hours of assistance in looking after the family after the baby is born. Contact them at 34 Elm Quay Court, Nine Elms Lane, London SW8 5DE, tel. 0171 498 2322.

A Private-Hospital Birth

If you want a private birth, look for a consultant you like and in whom you believe. A personal recommendation from someone you trust is the best method of finding the right person for you. If you go for your initial appointment and really dislike the consultant, change immediately.

PLUS POINTS
* You see the same consultant at every appointment and he or she will deliver your baby.
* You have your own room in the private wing of an NHS hospital or in a private hospital.
* Nappies, sheets etc. for the baby are provided for you.
* There is not so much pressure on bed space, so you can stay in hospital for longer than the average NHS patient if you wish.

MINUS POINTS
* The cost is around £3,000 or more (depending on where you deliver).
* Not all private hospitals have the facilities of a teaching hospital or a special-care unit.

Private Health Schemes and Birth

Do not assume that complications in pregnancy or assisted births are covered by your private health policy. Be sure to check if you are covered, and if not, what the maximum cost could be. If there are complications, it could prove astronomical. Older policies tend to be more generous than newer ones. Some doctors, however, offer a 'package' of a fixed price whatever the outcome.

The **Birth Unit, Hospital of St John and St Elizabeth**, 60 Grove End Road, London NW8 9NH, tel. 0171 286 5126, is host to the Active Birth list of the good and the great (for information on the Active Birth Movement, see page 42). Mothers have the choice of either consultant care, whereby all antenatal services are provided by an obstetrician (cost £3,200), or midwife care, whereby the majority of support is given by midwives (£2,500), though full medical back-up from obstetricians is available. Costs are exclusive of scans, antenatal screening or use of special-care facilities.

Tests and Screening

'Tests are not to frighten, they are there to inform.'
Cathy McCormick, Royal College of Midwives

Nearly every prospective mother worries about the health of her unborn baby. Tests should give you peace of mind that all is well. Because they are often regarded as 'routine', not too much time is allocated to explaining them. However, they are *not* routine for *you*: this is a special event in your life, so before you go ahead be sure that you are clear about:
- what you are being tested for;
- how you might deal with an unexpected result.

AIMS points out that 'You must be aware of the difficult choices you may have to make if a test result is unfavourable':

- Would you abort the baby if a test were to prove positive?
- Do you believe the tests?
- Would you be able to carry the baby to term and then deal with your grief if the baby were suffering from, say, a life-threatening illness?
- Would you prefer not to do the test?
- Will there be any point in having a test? Will it improve the outcome for you or your baby?

You must feel confident that it is better to have a test and know in advance than not know and carry the baby to term . . . It is a very individual matter, and you should take time to consider your feelings. Do not allow yourself to be rushed!

If you object to all or any of the tests you can refuse them. Similarly, if you are not offered a test that you want, you must ask for it (there may be a charge if it is not available on the NHS). Tests for inherited conditions are covered on pages 37–8.

If you are worried about the results of a test, or you have had difficulties with an earlier pregnancy, get an explanatory letter from your GP and get in touch with the **Harris Birthright Centre** at King's College Hospital, London, tel. 0171 346 3040/924 0714 or 0894), or ask your doctor or hospital to make the contact for you. The King's team specializes in advanced techniques for scanning and treating babies before birth. This service is free to all mothers having their baby within the NHS, and you will be seen within twenty-four hours.

Kypros Nicolaides has also opened the Fetal Medicine Centre at 8 Devonshire Place, London W1. It offers the latest in scanning and invasive testing. All profits go back into research into fetal medicine. Scans cost from £80.

If your doctor refuses to write a letter, or you are having a private birth and you want a thorough scan, you can be seen privately by experts at **Ultrasound Diagnostic Services**, 115 Harley Street, London W1, at a cost of £75 per scan. They prefer it if you allow them to write to your GP after the scan so that the results can be held with the rest of your notes.

Non-Invasive Tests

These will probably take place at each appointment and include urine tests, blood-pressure checks and measuring your weight to ensure that the pregnancy is progressing normally.

A number of blood tests are taken during antenatal visits; if you are unclear be sure to ask what you are being tested for.

Ultrasound Scans

Most women will be offered a scan during their pregnancy. Oil or jelly is squirted on to your tummy and a scanner is passed over it. Sound waves are transmitted to a screen to give a picture of the baby. You will probably be advised to drink a litre of water prior to the scan so you will be at bursting point by the time you are called. Spending time fiddling with clothes when you are desperate for the Ladies' is torture, so wear something simple. Take a spare pair of knickers, too, as these can get soaked with the jelly used by the scan operator. Ultrasound pictures fade with time, but Fotoscan/Shortland Prints can make long-lasting photographic-quality copies. Tel. 0161 485 7813 for details.

The scan can reveal whether you are expecting twins, if your due date is correct, and confirm that your baby is developing normally. A clear view of the baby's genital area will show the sex, but it can be difficult to be 100 per cent sure. Be aware of this if you are told the sex, though many hospitals will not share this information with you.

PLUS POINTS
* Non-invasive.
* Not proved to cause problems to the developing foetus.

MINUS POINTS
* A scan is only as good as the operator and his or her equipment. A poor operator could miss something vital.
* Can cause weeks of unnecessary anxiety if the reading is wrong or reveals something which turns out to be unimportant.

Nuchal Translucency Scan

This is a high-definition scan, performed at eleven to thirteen weeks, which is thought to be 80 per cent successful in screening for Down's syndrome. Operators measure a space at the back of the baby's neck. If it is over 2.5mm, it could indicate Down's. The test is available at large teaching hospitals or the **Harris Birthright Centre** (tel. 0171 346 3040). The test used to be free of charge, but demand is so great that most institutions now make a charge (around £40).

PLUS POINTS
* Non-invasive.
* Can detect other abnormalities.
* Not thought to harm the baby.

MINUS POINTS
* Still at the research stage.
* Will indicate the likelihood of Down's, but cannot tell you for sure.
* You will still be offered an amniocentesis or CVS if Down's is suspected.
* Criticized among obstetricians because many centres cannot achieve the same good results as those of the test's pioneers.
* Expensive.

Screening Tests

These *estimate* the chance of your baby having an abnormality. They do not screen for all possible abnormalities, nor do they give a definite diagnosis; instead they put you in a high- or low-risk category. The tests carry no risk to you or your baby and will (with a follow-up amniocentesis) help to detect 60 to 90 per cent Down's syndrome pregnancies. You will be offered a diagnostic test such as amniocentesis if you are considered high risk.

Most hospitals produce helpful leaflets explaining the tests, which should be given to you at your initial antenatal appointment.

AFP (Alpha Foetoprotein) Test

This screens for neural tube defects (NTDs) such as spina bifida and anencephaly. Performed at sixteen to eighteen weeks, it is available in most areas. High levels of AFP raise suspicion for an NTD.

> **PLUS POINT**
> * A simple blood test.
>
> **MINUS POINTS**
> * Can cause needless worries as in nine out of ten cases, raised AFP is attributable to an error in calculating your due date, twins or bleeding in early pregnancy.
> * Further tests such as an amniocentesis will still be offered if the baby's health is in any doubt.

Triple Test/Leeds/Bart's/Double Test

A blood test that measures 'markers' or biochemicals in the blood serum. It tells you whether your risk factor of having a baby with one of these conditions is higher or lower than normal for women of your age. It is performed at sixteen weeks and is available with most health authorities. Tests may be performed as early as thirteen weeks or as late as twenty-three weeks, but the ideal time for spina bifida and anencephaly detection using the Triple-Plus is between sixteen and eighteen weeks.

PLUS POINTS
* The most accurate form of non-invasive screening, especially the *Triple Test Plus*, a version which is performed three weeks earlier and is thought to detect around 15 to 20 per cent more Down's syndrome pregnancies than the double test. Kits are available on the NHS at some hospitals and fund-holding GPs. Otherwise you can obtain one for use by your doctor, price £88, from the University of Leeds, tel. 0113 234 4013. If you want further information on screening for Down's syndrome or Cystic Fibrosis, the Leeds Antenatal Screening Service can help.
* It may avoid unnecessary amniocentesis.

MINUS POINTS
* A low-risk result does not completely rule out the possibility of Down's syndrome.
* If there is thought to be a high risk, you will still need an amniocentesis, and much more likely than not it will turn out to be normal.

Diagnostic Tests

These indicate accurately whether your baby has a specific condition. They are invasive, which means that there is a risk of miscarriage.

Amniocentesis

In this test a needle is inserted into the amniotic fluid surrounding the baby and a sample is removed for analysis. The doctor will use an ultrasound scan to ensure that the needle does not touch the baby. It is usually performed at sixteen to eighteen weeks, sometimes earlier, though most centres consider amniocentesis before fifteen weeks too risky. Results come in after three weeks. This test is available to all expectant mothers.

> **PLUS POINT**
> * Very accurate in determining the sex of your baby and whether or not it has Down's syndrome or spina bifida.
>
> **MINUS POINTS**
> * The risk of miscarriage is 1 to 2 per cent.
> * There are at least 5,000 single-gene abnormalities, many of which it cannot detect, but special tests are available for some, e.g., cystic fibrosis.

CVS (Chorionic Villus Sampling)

This may be offered when there is a risk that the baby has a specific abnormality. It is the analysis of placental tissue, undertaken at ten to thirteen weeks. It can be done via the cervix, or using a similar procedure to amniocentesis. *You must insist on a highly experienced doctor performing this test: it could mean the difference between keeping your baby and a miscarriage.* If you are concerned about your hospital's facilities, ask them to refer you to places like the Harris Birthright Centre. The results take about ten days.

> **PLUS POINT**
> * It can give an earlier indication than an amniocentesis of chromosomal abnormalities.
>
> **MINUS POINTS**
> * Cannot detect all problems, e.g., spina bifida.
> * Babies can be damaged by the procedure.
> * Has a higher rate of miscarriage than amniocentesis, generally around 2 to 3 per cent.

Cordocentesis

Using ultrasound for guidance, a fine needle is inserted into the umbilical cord to take a sample of the baby's blood. This is cultured and tested for indications of a range of chromosomal disorders and blood diseases. It is performed at eighteen weeks, and results are given immediately or within two days. Cordocentesis is available at teaching hospitals and through private obstetricians.

> **PLUS POINT**
> * Fast results.
>
> **MINUS POINT**
> * At least a one in fifty chance of miscarriage.

Genetic Counselling

Genetic disorders are rare, but if there is a medical problem in your family that you think may be passed on to your unborn baby, seek advice immediately, preferably before conception. A huge variety of different medical conditions is caused by genetic inheritance, e.g. Duchenne Muscular Dystrophy, Cystic Fibrosis and Huntington's Chorea. Cleft lip and palate, an extra finger or congenital heart disease can also have a genetic link.

Your GP or midwife might refer you for genetic counselling if:
- a close relative has any of the above conditions, or Down's syndrome or other chromosomal abnormality;
- you already have a child with medical problems or learning difficulties, in which case you may want to know if the problem is genetic;
- you are on medication for conditions such as diabetes or epilepsy, or have had three or more miscarriages.

A genetic counsellor is a specially trained doctor or geneticist who will make detailed notes on the medical histories of the prospective parents and their families in an attempt to identify a defective gene. He/she will offer confidential, non-judgemental advice to parents before conception to allow them to make an informed choice, and if a problem is identified, the counsellor will explain all the options available.

Support groups exist for many genetic diseases. The counselling service closest to you will be best placed to tell you about local groups and national organizations. The best way to find these is through your GP.

The Genetic Interest Group (**GIG**), Farringdon Point, 29–35 Farringdon Road, London EC1M 3JB, tel. 0171 430 0090, is an alliance of charities and voluntary organizations for people affected by genetic disorders, and it can put individuals in touch with support groups and other local genetic services.

Antenatal Classes

The golden rule is: book your place as soon as possible. At their best, antenatal classes give you the information and support to transform a potentially stressful time into a joyous, fulfilling experience; at their worst, they can leave you feeling inadequate and unfit for parenthood. Whatever class you choose, you must remember that the teacher's values are her own, and you don't have to espouse them if they don't suit you. 'Natural childbirth' may be a solution for some, but the Almighty won't give you a black mark if you opt for every drug that medical science can offer.

Recent research has shown that preparation really does help you to cope with labour and its aftermath. However, do not put all your faith in exercises ensuring a pain-free delivery. They will work for some people and not for others, but at least give yourself that option. Even if the classes teach you little, they provide a valuable opportunity for you to make local friends who can be a source of practical and emotional support at a time when you badly need it.

You can always start off at a selection of classes before deciding which one suits you best. As well as the types listed below, you may find an excellent class that is exclusive to your area. Independent midwives sometimes give antenatal classes (see page 28).

If you can't get to an antenatal class, the Royal College of Midwives supply a range of free 'Informed Choice' leaflets on pregnancy topics, e.g. ultrasound and positions for labour. Tel. 0891 210400.

NHS Classes

These are held in hospitals and health centres, and start when you are around twenty-eight weeks' pregnant. Each course lasts six to eight weeks, and is free. Ask at your antenatal clinic for the course nearest to your due date. Often there is a choice of mothers' classes (including one session for partners) or couples' classes. (A partner in this context is the person who will be with you when you give birth. It does not necessarily have to be the baby's father.) You will receive advice on health, diet and exercise during pregnancy; the developing foetus and the mother's body changes; exercise and techniques to ease labour; signs of labour; when to go to hospital; what happens when you arrive; pain relief; feeding and caring for your baby.

PLUS POINTS
* Normally run by midwives or physiotherapists with first-hand knowledge of the hospital and its procedures.
* You become familiar with the hospital and its staff.

MINUS POINT
* Classes can be large and impersonal with little discussion time.

NCT Classes

These are held in the house of the teacher or a local member of the NCT (National Childbirth Trust). Starting when you are around twenty-eight weeks' pregnant, the course lasts six to nine weeks. Intensive 'crash courses' are also available in some areas. A course costs £30 to £90, depending on the branch and your ability to pay. Courses vary from area to area, but there is normally a choice of mothers' classes and mothers-and-partners' classes. The subjects covered are the same as those dealt with in NHS courses, but there is more of an accent on the emotional aspects of childbirth and the ways in which your partner can 'stand up' for you when you are in labour.

> **PLUS POINTS**
> * Small classes ensure that individual concerns can be addressed.
> * Relaxed, friendly atmosphere.
> * Provide access to all the NCT's services, including breastfeeding counsellors.
>
> **MINUS POINTS**
> * Can be expensive, though concessions are often available.
> * Classes may not be convenient for where you live.
> * Some teachers have a tendency to idealize childbirth and build up false expectations of easy deliveries.
> * You need to book your place very early – classes fill up quickly.

What is the NCT?

The **National Childbirth Trust**, Alexandra House, Oldham Terrace, London W3 6NH, tel. 0181 992 8637, is Britain's largest and most comprehensive voluntary organization devoted to education for childbirth. You do not have to be a member to attend the classes, though you will probably want to join once your lessons start. The NCT offers expert local assistance with breastfeeding and wonderful postnatal support.

Some people mistakenly believe that NCT stands for 'Natural' Childbirth Trust, and that members have to support childbirth without pain relief. On the contrary, the NCT's aim is to support all mothers and to assist them in making informed choices. Like any large organization, it does contain extremists, and in the NCT extremists are likely to be passionately opposed to clinical 'intervention' in a 'natural' birth. All the same, it would be a great shame to dismiss the NCT, as there are many benefits to be gained from it both before and after the birth of your baby. Many NCT volunteers seem to be direct descendants of Florence Nightingale, as you may well discover to your advantage on that awful evening alone at home with a screaming baby, the beginnings of mastitis and a desperate need for a postnatal sob in a sympathetic ear.

The local NCT newsletter will tell you about activities and services in your area. It will also put you in touch with a host of local mothers. The annual subscription is £12, or £18 to include their quarterly magazine, *New Generation*.

Cuidiu/Irish Childbirth Trust

Cuidiu (Irish for 'caring support') provides education and support for parents during pregnancy and through to adolescence. Parents with special needs are encouraged to attend and refresher courses are run for parents on subsequent pregnancies. Contacts: Dublin: Clair Allcut, tel. 01840 6489; Munster: Geraldine Daly, tel. 021 314705; Ulster 0762 849587.

Active Birth

Active Birth classes offer a holistic approach through exercise and relaxation techniques for pregnancy and birth, which aims to help mothers use their bodies to achieve as natural a birth as possible. Drugs and medical intervention during labour is usually discussed at the classes.

PLUS POINTS
* A way of meeting local pregnant mothers.
* Holistic approach to childbirth.

MINUS POINT
* May paint an unfairly rosy picture of natural birth so that mothers feel that they have 'failed' if labour requires medical intervention.

To find out more, send an SAE to the **Active Birth Movement**, 25 Bickerton Road, London N19 5JT, tel. 0171 561 9006.

Aquanatal Classes

Some local swimming baths or sports centres offer classes in which you exercise in water. Your community midwife or local hospital should be able to put you in touch with a teacher, but you should ensure that he or she is fully trained. In most cases you do not need to be able to swim. Classes cost around £3 a session, and are an excellent way of toning your body while you are pregnant.

Multiple Pregnancy

TAMBA

If you are expecting more than one baby, when you are four months' pregnant, contact **TAMBA**, the Twins and Multiple Births Association. Their help will be invaluable in supporting you through your pregnancy and afterwards. They can supply a comprehensive range of leaflets and books, too.

TAMBA will put you in touch with your local twins club, run by local mothers of multiples. Some twins clubs make a special point of organizing group events and teas so that you always have an outing to look forward to with mothers who understand what it's like coping with twins, triplets or more.

The TAMBA administrator, Gina Siddons, can be contacted via PO Box 30, Little Sutton, South Wirral L66 1TH, tel./fax 0151 348 0020.

The following specialist groups come under the TAMBA umbrella.
- The **One-Parent Families Group**, which aims to support families in which one parent is bringing up twins or triplets alone. They put families in touch with each other, and also

offer help with particular problems.
- The **Supertwins Group**, for families of triplets or more, run a contact scheme for information and moral support. A list of second-hand triple and quad buggies for sale is available from the group.
- The **Infertility Group** is for parents expecting twins, triplets or more as a result of fertility treatment. The group provides support from members with similar experience.
- The **Special Needs Group** assists families with special difficulties in bringing up multiples suffering from an illness or disability. A contact scheme puts parents in touch with others in a similar situation.
- The **Bereavement Support Group** offers support from parents who have suffered a similar loss, by phone and correspondence and through meetings. An annual memorial service is held.
- The **Health and Education Group** assesses the needs of families and provides information on the care of multiples. A free professional consultancy service is available for parents and professionals.

Choosing Your Medical Care

If you live in a large city, hold out for a midwife with experience of multiples and experience of helping mothers to breastfeed twins.

You need a big special-care unit so that the babies do not have to be separated. In some NHS hospitals, they will try hard to give you a room on your own.

Financial Assistance for Multiples

The government does not give extra financial help to families with multiples apart from the ordinary maternity payments and child benefit for each child (see Chapter 3). Your health visitor should know if the local council makes any special provision for mothers of triplets or more.

Shopping

In some areas, having a TAMBA membership card qualifies you for discounts at local shops, both smaller independent retailers and also large chain stores such as Children's World. It is well worth asking before you buy. For instance, you can get a 10 per cent reduction on shoes for all your children at Clark's shops. Your twins club will have a list of other helpful stores in your area.

TAMBA produces a leaflet called *Equipment and Clothing List for Newborn Multiples*, which you may find useful, particularly if you are trying to spread the cost of your purchases over a few months.

Some stores will deliver equipment. Londoners have the advantage of Nappy Express, tel. 0181 361 4040, for all baby and household goods. Boots operates a nappy-service and smaller local shops may also deliver.

Helpful Organizations

- **TAMBA Twinline**, tel. 01732 868000, is a national confidential listening, support and information service for all multiple-birth parents. It is open from 7 to 11 p.m. on weekdays and between 10 a.m. and 11 p.m. at weekends. If you would like to talk to experts in health, obstetrics, paediatrics etc., contact the TAMBA administrator for details. If you lose a twin through miscarriage, TAMBA can offer support in this situation too (see also Chapter 19).
- **The Multiple Births Foundation** is worth contacting if you have medical questions to ask. It is based at Queen Charlotte's Hospital, and welcomes inquiries from parents, health professionals or anyone caring for twins or more. They can be contacted during office hours at Queen

Charlotte's and Chelsea Hospital, Goldhawk Road, London W6 0X9, tel. 0181 740 3519.

Disability and Pregnancy

As a growing number of disabled women choose to have babies, more research and experience are contributing to improvements in care and support. Disabled mothers must find tremendous courage and determination to go through pregnancy so it seems particularly unfair that many feel they spend the whole time fighting the negative attitudes of others. The New Maternity Charter (see pages 17–18) is geared to improving this situation.

Antenatal Care

On discovering that you are pregnant, consider asking your GP the following type of questions.
- Can I park at the antenatal clinic?
- Is there wheelchair access?
- Can I have my appointments at home instead of going to the clinic or hospital?
- If I do have to go to hospital, is there a telephone number to ring to ensure that I am met on arrival by a volunteer or porter?
- Can hospital appointments be scheduled during quieter periods to give me extra time to come and go?

Ask the midwives or doctors who are looking after you if you can have a tour of the labour facilities to satisfy yourself that the appropriate equipment is available. Make sure they are aware of the nature of your disability and what your particular needs are. If you are going to have your baby in hospital, you might want to check, for example, that the beds have electric controls or that bathrooms are designed for wheelchair-users.

If you do not feel that you are getting a sympathetic, efficient service, go back to your GP and ask to be referred somewhere else. It makes all the difference if you have confidence in your carers.

Antenatal Classes

Ask your doctor or midwife:
- Can suitable exercise classes be arranged with an obstetric physiotherapist?
- Can I be given appropriate advice in drawing up my birth plan? (This is particularly important if there is a chance that you may be delivered by a midwife who does not know you.)
- Can breastfeeding advice be organized?
- Is there a local support group through which I can meet other disabled mothers?

Helpful Organizations

ParentAbility is a peer support network within the National Childbirth Trust which seeks to empower disabled people as parents and prospective parents. It runs two contact registers: one to help disabled parents to contact each other and the other for health professionals. Its services are free, although volunteers are welcome, as are any contributions to NCT funds. For details call the NCT's national office on 0181 992 8637.

The network publishes *The ParentAbility Resource List*, an 84-page guide to pregnancy, birth and parenthood, at £5.40 including post and packing. It can be obtained from NCT Maternity sales, tel. 0141 633 5552, fax. 0141 633 5677. Visually impaired people can call 01744 451215 for a free taped version.

There is also a quarterly magazine, *Disability, Pregnancy and Parenthood International*, for professionals and parents worldwide to exchange information and experience. Subscription rates are £12 per annum (reduced to £7.50 for ParentAbility members) in the UK. For further information and a sample copy, contact Arrowhead Publications, 1 Chiswick Staithe, London W4 3TP, tel. 0181 994 0896.

Equipment

Equipped is a joint initiative between ParentAbility and a number of organizations concerned with meeting the equipment needs of disabled people. Both disabled parents and their health professionals often have difficulty in finding appropriate equipment, and Equipped should have the answers to any queries. If you need equipment to be adapted for you get in touch well in advance. Telephone Lisa Nichols on 01895 675630 for further information.

In addition to its main campaigning work, **RADAR**, the organisation that fights for the rights of disabled people, offers a rather useful sideline: second-hand equipment, which is advertised for sale in the *RADAR Bulletin*. You can advertise your own equipment for £5. Contact Claire Skinner at RADAR on 0171 250 3222.

Parents With Learning Disabilities

The British Institute of Learning Disabilities (**BILD**) publishes a series of five booklets entitled *I want to be a good parent*, tackling issues from what it is like to be a parent to the love children need. They cost £10 each, including postage and packing, or £37.50 for the series. Telephone 01562 850251 for further details.

2   Taking Care of Yourself

Your Diet

Your doctor or midwife is the best person to give you dietary advice to suit your particular requirements. There is normally a variety of free booklets in the doctor's surgery and antenatal clinic advising you on how to eat healthily. If you cannot find such leaflets there, the **Centre for Pregnancy Nutrition** will send you a free information pack. Ring 0114 242 4084 between 10 a.m. and 2 p.m. to speak to a dietician; at other times leave your name and address on the answerphone.

Aim for a diet that is low in fatty, sugary foods, e.g., ready-made biscuits, cakes, pastries and fried food, because these are low in vitamins and minerals as well as being high in calories. Try to eat:

- cereals, potatoes, bread, pasta, rice – particularly the 'high-fibre' varieties, e.g., wholemeal bread and pasta, wholegrain breakfast cereals and brown rice;
- fruit and vegetables;
- meat, fish and vegetarian alternatives, e.g., nuts and pulses;
- milk and dairy products, especially low-fat varieties.

All pregnant women are now strongly recommended to take a folic acid supplement from conception to the end of the first three months of pregnancy. This greatly reduces the risk of neural-tube defects in your baby. If you want to take folic acid before you are pregnant, your doctor will usually give you two months' supply. For more information about folic acid, ring the

Folic Acid Helpline, part of the **Medical Advisory Service**, tel. 0181 994 9874, which operates between 2 p.m. and 10 p.m. from Monday to Friday, or the Pregnancy Nutrition Helpline on the same number.

If you are told to take an iron supplement and this makes you constipated, take Floradix, which contains iron extracted from plants. This is available in liquid or tablet form at £6.89 for 250ml or £5.50 for a month's tablets. It is expensive, but preferable to the alternative.

Tips for a Healthy Diet

- If you cannot stand brown bread, look for the new types of white bread with added fibre.
- Buy fresh vegetables in small quantities and eat them immediately – storage reduces the vitamin content. Frozen vegetables have the same vitamin content as fresh ones.
- Dried and canned vegetables have a reduced vitamin content.
- Raw vegetables contain higher levels of vitamins than cooked ones.
- Steaming or microwaving vegetables retains higher levels of vitamins than boiling them.
- If you have to boil vegetables, use only the smallest amount of water – some vitamins leak into the water. Try to reuse the cooking water in other dishes, e.g., stocks and sauces.
- Processed fruit juices lack fibre, although they do contain vitamins and minerals.
- Cut visible fat off all meat.
- Remove the skin from chicken.
- Grill sausages, bacon, etc., rather than frying them.
- Avoid processed meat products such as sausage rolls and pork pies as they are very fatty.
- Low-fat cheeses and yoghurt provide as much calcium as the standard alternatives.

Pregnancy

- UHT milk does not have as many vitamins as fresh milk.
- Oven chips or home-made thick-cut ones contain less fat than fine-cut frozen varieties.
- Avoid foods in breadcrumbs and batter.
- Look for low-fat versions of foods.
- Try to eat fresh fruit instead of pudding or chocolates at the end of a meal. Bananas may suppress cravings for fatty, sugary foods.
- Glucose, sucrose, maltose and dextrose are all sugars – be aware of them on labels.

★★★ Star buys ★★★

Boots fortified milk drink (strawberry or banana flavour) includes folic acid, calcium, thiamin (vitamin B1), riboflavin (B2) and B12. Price: 55p.

Food Safety

What to Avoid

- **Prepared foods.** Ready-roasted chickens and prepared meals from the chilled cabinet could harbour listeria, toxoplasmosis or salmonella. Listeria is a bacterium that can cause miscarriage, usually in the second trimester.
- **Raw eggs.** Eggs should be eaten only when both yolk and white are cooked until solid. Home-made mayonnaise should be avoided. Shop-bought branded mayonnaise is safe as it is made with pasteurized eggs.
- **Certain dairy products.** Mould-ripened soft cheeses, e.g., Brie and Camembert; blue-veined cheeses such as Stilton or Danish blue; unpasteurized cows' milk; soft ice-cream from machines. There is a risk of listeria with all of these.
- **Liver or liver-based foods such as pâté.** These contain high levels of vitamin A which could endanger the health of your baby.

- **Raw or undercooked meat.** Especially during the barbecue season, be very careful that meat is cooked right through. Otherwise you run the risk of contracting toxoplasmosis, which can severely damage your baby.
- **Processed foods.** If you must buy them, compare the ingredients of similar products to help you to choose the healthiest brand. Ingredients are listed in order of the percentage of the product they represent. The higher up the list, the larger the amount of the ingredient the product contains. So if the label says 'Apples, water, sugar', there will be more apples than water and more water than sugar.
- **Caffeinated drinks.** Tea, coffee, Coca-Cola, all contain caffeine. It is thought that they may affect birth weight if consumed in excessive quantities (over five cups of normal-strength coffee, ten cups of tea or eight cans of Coke per day).
- **Alcohol.** In regular, large doses, alcohol can cause foetal alcohol syndrome – low birth weight and permanent brain damage. Do not get tipsy or drunk during pregnancy.

Fish

A study of the diets of pregnant women in the Faroe Isles revealed that eating fish up to three times a week can improve the size of babies (*Journal of Epidemiology and Community Health*, 1993). You may wish to avoid the more exotic varieties – especially if you are on holiday in a hot climate.

Food Preparation

To avoid infection, always cook meat thoroughly and wash your hands and all surfaces and utensils which have been in contact with raw meat. Wash all fruit and vegetables well and discard anything remotely mouldy.

To ensure that your fridge keeps food in perfect condition:
- Keep it at a temperature of between 0 and 5 degrees C (32 and 41 degrees F). Fridge thermometers, which cost around

£2.95, are sold at John Lewis stores or Boots. A mercury thermometer is not suitable as it will break. The thermostat inside the fridge does not show the temperature.
- Do not overfill the fridge as this prevents it from operating efficiently.
- Let hot food cool before putting it into the fridge.
- Cover all foods so that they cannot drip or otherwise contaminate other items.
- Do not keep food beyond its 'use-by' date.
- Do not leave bags of groceries in a warm car. The temperature could encourage the growth of harmful bacteria.

Combating Morning Sickness

If you are vomiting a lot do not clean your teeth afterwards. Use a fluoride mouthwash instead. Vomiting and then brushing your teeth erodes tooth enamel.

Eat a dry biscuit or a piece of dry toast before getting up in the morning. Ginger biscuits are often recommended, as is sucking on peeled ginger root or eating crystallized ginger. Snack on dry foods and substitute coffee with peppermint tea and ginger drinks such as ginger ale. Isotonic fizzy 'sports' drinks replace fluids and minerals and may make you feel better.

If these don't work:
- homoeopaths often recommend ipecacuanha, but check with a qualified homoeopath before taking anything.
- Try travel-sickness bands, available from the chemist. Worn on both wrists they can counteract many forms of nausea.
- Acupuncture may help, but check with your GP first and only go to a recommended practitioner (see the section on Complementary Medicines and Therapies in Chapter 6).

Further Advice

The **Food Safety Directorate** produces a series of colourful booklets called *Foodsense*. Titles include *Keeping Food Cool and*

Safe (pb1649), *Food Safety* (pb0551) and *Healthy Eating* (pb0550). Contact Foodsense, London SE99 7TT, tel. 0645 556000 for your free copies. The **Centre for Pregnancy Nutrition** has the booklets too.

Healthy Eating For You and Your Baby, written by three experts from the Centre for Pregnancy Nutrition, published by Pan, costs £5.99 in paperback (ISBN 0 330 33755 6) and is available through Book Service by Post Ltd on 0162 4675137 or from bookshops.

Medicines and Pregnancy

Be careful

- Never use left-over medicines, and never try a new medicine while you are pregnant.
- Don't pick up a repeat prescription without informing your doctor that you are pregnant.
- Always mention to your pharmacist that you are pregnant when purchasing *any* medicine.
- Recreational drugs such as marijuana should be avoided.
- Avoid skin creams with steroids.

Drugs Used in Pregnancy

Pain relief. Paracetamol may be allowed – ask your GP. Avoid aspirin as it can cause foetal abnormalities or bleeding.

Coughs and colds. Avoid cold remedies. Take hot lemon and honey or camomile tea with honey instead.

Tummy upsets. Drink plenty of fluids. A hot-water bottle on your tummy can be soothing. Antacids are often prescribed.

Antibiotics. Most penicillins are fine as long as you do not suffer an allergic reaction to this drug. But there are still many that are contraindicated. Always remind your doctor that you are pregnant before he prescribes something for you.

Asthma inhalers. Inhalers can normally be used, but asthma should be monitored carefully throughout pregnancy.

Epilepsy drugs. Some drugs can harm the foetus, so seek specialist advice, but never stop medication unless directed to do so by your doctor, as untreated epilepsy also carries a risk of damage. Safe alternatives can always be prescribed.

Insulin for diabetes. Your needs will change during pregnancy. Check with your doctor.

Anti-nausea/sickness. Treatment is administered only for serious problems, and the range of drugs used is very limited. See pages 120–27 for some natural remedies.

Immunizations. Vaccines which contain a 'live' virus should be avoided during pregnancy, especially the rubella (German measles) vaccination. It is not advisable to take malaria tablets.

Antidepressants. Check with your doctor before you are pregnant, as you may need to change from one brand to another before trying to conceive.

A note on smoking

Smoking or being in a constantly smoky atmosphere can be seriously detrimental to your unborn baby's health. Your GP may run a Stop Smoking clinic that you can attend. Otherwise, Smokers Quitline, on 0171 487 3000, can offer advice. They are open seven days a week.

Beauty During Pregnancy

'Using stretch-mark cream is like putting your socks on in the morning and expecting them to be absorbed into your legs by the afternoon.'
Midlands-based dermatologist

Some women spend nine months of pregnancy waiting to 'bloom' but their hormones have already decided otherwise: dry skin, rashes, itches and stretch marks are the fate of the unlucky few. Here are some beauty products designed to deal with typical minor irritations.

Hair

If you are doing a lot of swimming during pregnancy and you find that it is harming your hair, look out for UltraSwim Protective Shampoo and Conditioner. Both cost £2.85 for 236ml from Boots and large chemists.

Thrush and Cystitis

Popular remedies include Canestan (£9 for 50g) or Vagisil (£3.29 for 30g). For cystitis, either Cystemme (£3.59), Cystopurin (£3.61) or Cynalon (£3.99) should help.

Soreness and Piles

Nipple creams such as Lansinoh (from £3.50), available mail order from Egnell Ameda, tel. 01823 336362, will soothe a range of conditions.

If you are suffering from piles you can get Anusol in either cream or suppository form. The latter is better for internal piles. Twelve cost £3.95. Hackle's Derma Cure moist toilet tissues are designed for women suffering from piles, sore stitches or skin irritations (£2.25 from chemists and supermarkets).

Skin

Lynne Sanders of Cosmetics à la Carte says, 'Whatever changes you see in your skin, the most important thing is to clean it thoroughly – especially if you live in a city. People look at their face and think it is their skin that is dry and flaky, but it may be a thin layer of dirt. Cleanse your face as you usually do, but in addition, once a week, use an exfoliating or refining mask such as Avon's Revitalizing Face Mask (£2.29 for 75ml).

You may find that bubble bath causes irritation such as thrush or cystitis, but old-fashioned bath salts should be fine. Otherwise, look out for the Simple range – soap is 49p, shower gel £2.39 – or Wash E45 or Bath E45, both £3.15.

If someone wants to give you a present, you might ask for Crabtree & Evelyn's Revitalizing Mineral Muscle Soak (£12.50), which turns your water bright turquoise with its combination of Epsom and Dead Sea salts, to ease fatigue, and peppermint oil, sea algae and camomile to soften the skin.

Vaseline is the beauty jack-of-all-trades for pregnant women. It is hypoallergenic, it lubricates and softens dry skin, it can give temporary relief to external haemorrhoids and scaling due to psoriasis and it removes eye make-up (£1.29 for 50ml).

Itching

Itchy skin is occasionally a sign of a condition called obstetric cholestasis. This is rare but controllable, so always tell your doctor if you are feeling itchy. Wear cotton clothes and wash frequently to stop sweat building up. If putting a bag of frozen peas over the itch does not help, a cream might. Ask your pharmacist.

If you suddenly become itchy, you may have developed an allergy to a particular food or beauty product. Avon's Intense Moisture Body Lotion, suitable for all skin types, is hypoallergenic and soothing. Freephone 0800 663 664 to arrange a visit from your nearest representative.

Around 70 per cent of pregnant women suffer from red spots and thread veins. You can cover them with make-up and hamper their growth by avoiding extremes of temperatures, very hot drinks and spicy foods. If you are concerned about looking red in the face, try the Body Shop's Colourings Colour Balance Fluid in green (£3.95) or their green Colour Balance Translucent Powder (£2.95), which you apply over your own translucent powder. Boots No. 7 products are fragrance-free and hypoallergenic. They sell a light diffusing tinted moisturizer for £4.50.

Brown patches (chloasma)

These can appear on the skin, often on the cheeks, forehead or around the eyes. They usually fade in the months following the birth. If they do not, your doctor can prescribe a bleaching agent – but only after the pregnancy. It is quite an art to disguise chloasma without looking overmade-up, but Dermablend products, available from department stores and chemists, should provide good cover. Alternatively, try sandwiching Colourings Extra Cover from the Body Shop, £3.25, between two layers of foundation.

Sun makes chloasma worse. Use a high-protection sunblock such as Estee Lauder Advanced Suncare Sunblock SPF25. You can wear make-up over it.

Breakouts

Spots can be a problem, but even if you look like a Dalmatian, you cannot take medication unless it is prescribed by your doctor. Clarins Gel Blemish Corrector (£10) will take the heat out of spots. Apply this before going to bed. During the day hide them with a concealer such as Colourings Extra Cover Concealer, £3.25 from the Body Shop.

Make-up

If you look pale and exhausted in the summer, use bronzing powder. The Body Shop's Colourings Tinted Bronzing Powder (£4.40 for 12g) is good value, as is Max Factor Natural Brush-On Satin Blush, which comes in eight shades, at £3.99. In winter use creamy blushers in coppery tones. Shadowy eyes can be rectified by Cosmetics à la Carte's Secret Light (£15). This is a light-reflecting product designed to counteract shadows and redness.

Cosmetics à la Carte will send you samples of their products so that you can try before you buy. Telephone 0171 622 2318 for details.

Stretch Marks

Nothing can prevent stretch marks, but you may find that Avon's Total Coverage Concealer (£3.79, available in three shades) disguises them. It is water-resistant, a sunscreen and is designed to cover all marks, blemishes and bruises.

Bad Back

If your GP or midwife can offer no help, telephone for the Back Shop catalogue (0171 935 9120), which carries a range of supportive chairs as well as office seating, work-station and other office equipment. You can also visit the shop, at 24 New Cavendish street, London W1M 7LH.

Feet

If your feet can take you as far as the high street, both Boots and the Body Shop stock a range of products to soothe and revitalize tired legs and feet. The Body Shop's Cooling Leg Gel (60ml for 90p) is formulated for pregnant women. If you cannot face the walk, try a Foot Soothing Mask (£4.95 for 100g plus postage and packing) from the Clay Company (tel. 0151 733 6900).

Mail order

If you prefer to contemplate new beauty routines from your armchair, you can ring for the following catalogues: Molton Brown By Mail (0171 625 6550); Yves Rocher's Green Book of beauty (0181 845 1222).

Maternity Bras

'If you insist on wearing an underwired bra any longer, your breasts will end up round your ankles.'
Doctor to woman five months pregnant

Bras for Pregnancy

It is being pregnant which changes your breasts, not breastfeeding. During pregnancy your breasts will get bigger and heavier as the milk-producing cells and ducts develop. Anticipate an overall increase, in both bust size and cup size, of about two bra sizes. For example, if you normally take a 34B, you will probably need a 38D. Wearing a good bra both before and after your baby is born is probably the best way to preserve your shape, at least cosmetically: bras are considerably more effective and cheaper than pots of bust-firming gel or surgery.

Although a few women do feel comfortable without a bra during pregnancy, most find the increased weight and size of their breasts cry out for good support. You can buy a special maternity bra (from around £10) if you wish, but this is not vital: comfort and fit are the most important factors. For many women this means a normal medium- or firm-support bra, or perhaps a good sports bra. Hugely popular with pregnant women is the Marks & Spencer Sports Bra (model 0518) at £9.

A good bra for pregnancy or breastfeeding:
- provides a firm shelf of support under the cup-line;
- covers the breast well so that no flesh bulges over the top or out at the sides;
- has no sharp edges or wires to dig into the breast;
- has some spare space around your nipplees;
- has wide, non-elastic straps;
- supports you at the back as well as the front, yet does not feel restrictive;
- does not ride up your back – when trying a bra keep it on

for a few minutes and waggle your arms to make sure;
- has plenty of size adjustment at the back to accommodate growth (Emma Jane and Mava sell extenders for around £1.25 if you grow more than you have anticipated);
- has a high cotton content – pregnancy and lactation can be sweaty times;
- unfastens – and refastens – discreetly and easily for feeding, ideally needing only one hand.

It is essential to be measured properly, around the bra you are already wearing. You need a store which has:
- a wide selection;
- trained staff;
- changing rooms.

Where to shop

Star buys are most likely to be found in John Lewis stores. They have well-trained fitters and a selection of brands: look out for the very good, but not cheap, Royce, Emma Jane and Triumph labels. Mothercare and Boots offer a range of suitable bras but as they only sell their own brands you may feel your choice is limited. There are trained fitters in many of these stores.

The NCT trains bra-fitters who work from home. They sell the excellent Mava range of bras, plus nightwear and other items. Phone your local branch to find out more.

Different brands suit differently shaped women. Or, to quote one retailer, 'A Triumph lady is not an Emma Jane lady.' Try on lots of bras before making your selection; do not 'make do'.

If you are confined to your home, or rushed into hospital, and somebody else has to shop for you, you can measure yourself as follows. First, put on a bra, then run a tape measure round your ribcage just under your breasts, holding it firmly but not pulling it tight. Ask someone else to hold the tape so that you can put your arms by your sides. If the measurement is an even number, add 6in; if it is odd add 5.

For example, 29in + 5 = 34. This is your bra size.

Measure round your breasts where they are fullest. The difference between this measurement and the previous one determines your cup size.

Bra size + 1 inch = B cup;   Bra size + 4 inch = DD cup;
Bra size + 2 inch = C cup;   Bra size + 5 inch = E cup.
Bra size + 3 inch = D cup;

It must be stressed that there is no substitute for being properly measured by a trained fitter and trying on a number of different designs.

You will find that you may try six or seven bras which are marked the same size but probably only one or two designs will really fit you.

Mothernature run a national mail order service, and carry a variety of bras ranging to a J fitting.

Sleep Bras

Sleep bras are often recommended for women with larger breasts to provide light support at night during pregnancy and breastfeeding. Choose one which opens easily or pushes well out of the way for night-time feeding. It must be able to support you without putting pressure on any part of your breast – a seam digging into you could block milk ducts and cause mastitis. High-street brands are available from £7, but the Mava Night-Time, at £9.50, is worth the extra cost.

Nursing Bras

A good nursing bra is invaluable. Wait until you are at least thirty-six weeks' pregnant to be fitted – by this time your baby may be lying lower in your body, allowing more room for accurate measurement. You will need two, ideally three, nursing bras. Expect to pay anything from £10 to £20. Buy the best you can afford. There are three types of nursing bra:

Front-Opening Bras. Each cup fastens to a centre band by means of a row of rather fiddly hooks and eyes. However, this is the most supportive type of bra and is ideal for women with larger breasts.

Zip-Opening Bras. Each cup unzips for feeding. This type of bra is also wonderfully supportive, and it has the advantage of exposing each breast completely so that there is no restrictive material lying across it. One-handed use is possible with practice, but watch you don't catch your breast in the zip.

Drop-Cup Bras. The cups hook on and off each shoulder strap. Make sure that the inner frame of the cup does not put pressure on the breast during feeding. Some models have small retaining ribbons to prevent wandering straps. This bra requires two-handed operation, but is still fairly discrete to open and close.

Maternity Clothes

It is no longer true that maternity wear makes you look like a mobile armchair. Simple, stylish clothes are available to everyone in Britain by mail order as well as from specialist shops. Whatever you buy will not be a waste of money, as long as it's comfortable – it will have at least one season's hard wear.

Maternity wear sizes correspond to your pre-pregnancy size. So if you are normally a size 14, buy that unless your bust has increased by over 3in.

Bottoms

If you are just going to buy one item, go for a skirt or leggings. You will need to wear loose-fitting items of clothing for a few weeks after the birth as your tummy may take a while to return to its normal size. Most maternity leggings, worn back to front, look great on post-pregnant women.

Taking Care of Yourself

Squat down to check that leggings fit neatly over your bottom and don't gape. Ensure that there is space for your bottom and thighs to swell as well as your tummy.

Maternity leggings at Dorothy Perkins start at £9.99. If you want to splash out, the Formes mail order catalogue (tel. 0171 737 5211) has skirts starting at £33. Their ribbed-panel system is comfortable on your tummy and the skirt will look neat and tailored.

C&A are planning a range of leggings and knitted skirts in navy, black, natural and pastel colours ranging from £7.99 to £9.99.

Tops

If you like the 'outsize' look, you can get ex-hire dinner jackets at second-hand shops and formal-wear stores such as Youngs. Prices vary from shop to shop. You might be able to pick one up in a charity shop for £5 or so. Cream dinner jackets look particularly splendid.

Large, loose tops look best with straight skirts, while long, straight tops are more flattering with full skirts. Waistcoats and cardigans can have a slimming effect.

Working Wardrobes

If you need to buy a suit for work, mail-order firms Blooming Marvellous, Formes and Jojo have a good selection. The Blooming range, made in Ireland and available from maternity-wear shops and department stores, offers a wonderful choice of separates which can be mixed and matched to provide both a working and a weekend wardrobe. Leggings start at around £25, which may seem expensive, but you are paying for quality and they will still look fine after the baby is born. Call 00 353 1 454 3366 for stockists, or 0171 436 1059 for UK inquiries.

Underwear

If your legs are not giving you too much trouble, start off with ordinary extra-large tights, turned back to front so that the back panel covers your bump. If you need some serious support, the best maternity support tights are Dr Scholl Lite Legs Maternity (£4.50). They soothe tired legs and help prevent varicose veins.

Hose by Post offer top-quality support stockings. Call 01535 667535 for their brochure.

Maternity suspender belts (£15.99) are available from Emma Jane mail order on 0181 599 3004, or try 0141 647 8106. If you are carrying twins or more, you will probably find that a Kumfibump (£39.99) offers tremendous comfort and support. This is a one-piece stretch-lace garment that supports your bump and your back. Call Krucial Kids, 0181 550 4935 for mail order.

Mothercare Support Briefs (£15, sizes 10–20) are also designed to support aching lower backs.

Swimwear

Avoid excessive ruching: it is unflattering, and the swimsuit will balloon when you are in the water. Swimwear mail-order stockists include NCT Maternity Sales (tel. 0141 633 5552); Jojo (0171 352 5156); Emma Jane (0181 599 3004) and Mothercare.

Hiring occasion wear and wedding dresses

Hiring these expensive items is becoming increasingly popular. Many independent retailers who stock maternity wear now offer a hire service, e.g., some branches of Bumpsadaisy.

Maternity Wear by Mail Order

Mail-order catalogues are free. The great advantage of 'armchair shopping' is that you do not have to squeeze yourself into a changing room designed for non-pregnant women. Most catalogues offer an automatic refund if you return pristine goods within ten days of delivery in their original wrapping with a copy of the invoice. Remember to retain proof of postage. There are a number of specialist mail-order firms.

Becoming (tel. 01793 537905) offer underwear, nightwear, casual wear and occasion wear. They will make and alter clothes, too. **Blooming Marvellous** (tel. 0181 391 4822) produce a lively, extensive catalogue full of good-value items for work and relaxation. They also have a shop, in Barnet, Hertfordshire (near the M25, junction 24), tel. 0181 441 5582. For underwear, there is **Emma Jane** (tel. 0181 599 3004).

Formes (tel. 0171 820 3456) provide an expensive French catalogue, small but exquisite, featuring work, casual and evening wear. They have two shops in London (tel. 0171 584 3337). Another upmarket company is **Great Expectations** (tel. 0171 581 4886). Their catalogue includes a little black dress for those who are not quite so little. The shop number is 0171 584 2451.

If you yearn for a more traditional look, **From Here to Maternity** (tel. 0191 386 5918) complete with a made-to-measure service, is for you. They also have a hire service.

If you love silk, the small catalogue from **Labour of Love** (tel. 01428 608345) could be right up your street. A shop is open off the A3 south of Guildford, but ring if you want to visit. They will open after-work hours if required.

The **Mothercare** catalogue (price 50p), available in their stores, includes home-shopping details. Their range includes nightshirts and knickers and other bits and pieces to take into hospital, and there is an extensive range of baby equipment.

Other maternity mail-order services are supplied by **JoJo** (tel. 01428 608345) and **Pregnant Pause** (tel. 01827 720435).

Travelling When Pregnant

Air Travel

Although most forms of transport are perfectly safe for a pregnant woman, it is vital to check with your doctor if you intend to fly beyond twenty-eight weeks of pregnancy. It is also important to consult your doctor if you are taking a long-haul flight, where your body has to cope with the cabin pressure for much longer. Make sure that you stretch your legs and walk about once an hour.

The increased pressure in an aircraft can cause fluid retention, which in turn puts extra pressure on the abdomen. If you have blood-pressure problems, they can be exacerbated by air travel.

Pregnant women are often allowed priority boarding and to jump the queue at check-in. Both British Airways and Virgin Atlantic recommend that you speak out if you want assistance: your pregnancy may not be obvious to the airline staff.

Travel Insurance

Most travel-insurance policies will cover the cost of your holiday if you need to cancel it and will meet medical expenses incurred overseas. This is normally straightforward, but if you are pregnant you need to be aware of the following:

- Most insurance companies will not pay for medical expenses incurred in connection with pregnancy or childbirth if you are twenty-eight weeks' pregnant or more. You are therefore unlikely to be compensated if you have to cut short your holiday after the twenty-eight-week mark.
- A claim is invalid if you travel against your doctor's advice, so check with your doctor before you book your travelling arrangements, even if you are less than twenty-eight weeks' pregnant.

- If you want to cancel your holiday but you knew that you were pregnant when you booked, you are entitled to a refund only if your doctor has advised that it would be unwise for you to travel.
- If you want to cancel a holiday booked before you discovered you were pregnant, and you will be over twenty-eight weeks into the pregnancy when you travel, you should be able to get a full refund on deposits for both your family and yourself. You will need a doctor's certificate giving your expected date of delivery and confirming that you did not know you were pregnant when you booked your holiday.
- If you decide not to go on an exotic holiday you have already booked because the jabs required might hurt the baby, you may not qualify for a refund of your deposit.

Car Travel

The Comfitum seatbelt guide, a padded accessory that 'guides' the seatbelt under your bump and prevents it pressing on your tummy, costs £14.99 at the Early Learning Centre and independent nursery shops.

Eating on Holiday

Pregnant women on holiday in countries where the water is unsafe to drink should avoid:
- shellfish;
- food which has been made in advance and reheated;
- water and milk which has not been boiled;
- fresh ice-cream – buy reputable, factory-made brands;
- unpeeled fruit and vegetables – peel and wash thoroughly in safe water before eating;
- food from street vendors.

3 Law and Finance

Pregnant Women at Work

Antenatal Appointments

You are entitled to attend your antenatal appointments without any deductions being made from your pay. This also applies to parentcraft and relaxation classes, although you may need a letter from your doctor, midwife or health visitor to explain these to your employer.

You should let your employer know the times you are likely to be absent. Your employer has the right to see your appointment card and a certificate from your doctor or midwife stating that you are pregnant if he or she wishes.

If you are not given the time off to attend classes, you can make a claim to an industrial tribunal within three months of the date of the appointment.

There are circumstances in which an employer may reasonably refuse to allow an employee time off for antenatal appointments, e.g. if you work part time, but there has to be agreement on both sides.

Health and Safety at Work

Special rules apply for women who are pregnant, those who have given birth within six months and those who are breastfeeding.

You must notify your employer in writing of any potential risks, in order to enforce the rules. Once alerted, your employer must analyse the potential risks and do what he or she can to remove or reduce them by amending your working hours or conditions, by offering you alternative work or by suspending you on full pay until it is safe for you to return to work. If you unreasonably refuse to do different work you lose the right to be suspended on full pay.

If you work at night and your doctor advises you to stop on health grounds, you are entitled to work during the day instead or to be suspended on full pay if your employer cannot find you suitable alternative work. You will need a medical certificate.

Maternity Leave

Fourteen weeks' maternity leave is available to all women employees who work while they are pregnant. Your non-wage-related contractual benefits (for example, holiday entitlement and company car) must be maintained: only your pay will differ (see the information on benefits on pages 72–6 for details).

To qualify
- You must tell your employer in good time. Notice should be given not less than twenty-one days before the date on which you intend to commence your maternity leave.
- You do not need to have worked a certain number of hours or for the same company for a specific period of time.
- When you are six months' pregnant you must give form MAT B1 to your employer.

Returning to Work
- You do not need to give notice if you are going back to work at the end of fourteen weeks. If you are returning early, you must give seven days' notice in writing.
- You are not allowed to work for two weeks after the baby is born, so if your baby is born so late that your fourteen weeks

have run out, your leave is extended by two additional weeks.
- Your employer can delay your return for four weeks, but if so he or she must tell you why.
- If a strike or interruption to work interferes with your ability to tell your employer that you want to go back, you can delay your return for up to twenty-eight days after the end of the interruption.
- If an employer writes to you after eleven weeks of your maternity leave asking for confirmation that you will be going back to work, you must respond in writing within fourteen days or your right to return is cancelled.
- You can delay your return, once, by up to four weeks if you are sick and have a medical certificate. If you do so you must notify your employer and make an agreement with her before the date that you are expected back.

Extended Maternity Absence

This is available to women who have worked continuously for the same employer for not less than two years at the beginning of the eleventh week before the expected week of childbirth. (This extension may not be open to women who work in a company which employs five people or fewer.)

In addition to the standard fourteen weeks available to all working women, you are allowed a further twenty-nine weeks' unpaid leave after the birth. This starts from the beginning of the week in which your baby is born. Twenty-one days before you go back you must give notice of the day you are returning. This is called the notified date of return.

To qualify
- You must give notice in good time that you are pregnant.
- You must inform your employers in writing that you intend to return to work after the birth.

If you are dismissed because you are pregnant or on maternity leave

Your employer is breaking the law if he or she dismisses you or selects you for redundancy because you are pregnant or on maternity leave. The length of time you have held your job or whether you work part-time is irrelevant.

If your employer dismisses you while you are pregnant or on maternity leave, he or she must automatically give you a written statement explaining why. If you think your pregnancy is the reason for your dismissal, see your trade union representative or solicitor, or visit your Citizens' Advice Bureau. Your claim against your employer must be presented to an industrial tribunal before the end of three months. (It is worth noting that in this instance the three months is up a day earlier than you might expect. If, for example, you were dismissed on 2 March, the application would have to be submitted by 1 June, not 2 June.)

If you are sacked, your hours are cut or you are demoted, or you think that you have been discriminated against in any way because you are pregnant or have had a baby, you can claim that you have been discrimated against because you are a woman. No qualifying period of employment is required in the case of sexual discrimination, but you will need legal advice and claims must be made within three months of the last act of discrimination.

This section was written with assistance from Jane Richards and Tania Stevenson, Frere Cholmely Bischoff, Solicitors, 4 John Carpenter Street, London EC4Y 0NH, tel. 0171 615 8000.

For information on maternity rights contact the Maternity Alliance, 45 Beech Street, London EC2P 2LX (tel. 0171 588 8582), or send an sae for their free leaflet 'Pregnant At Work'.

Benefits

Your employer is obliged by law to grant you the following maternity benefits as a minimum. Some companies are more generous than others, and you may find that your own terms are more advantageous.

Statutory Maternity Pay (SMP)

This is a weekly payment for women who remain employed during pregnancy, even if they do not go back to work after the baby is born. It begins when you start your maternity leave and will normally be paid in the same way as your salary or wages are usually paid, weekly or monthly. Eleven weeks before the birth is the earliest time you can opt for your SMP to start – it is up to you to decide how late in the pregnancy you want to work.

To qualify
- You must have worked for the same employer continuously for at least twenty-six weeks by the end of the fifteenth week before the week the baby is due.
- You must still be in your job at the fifteenth-week mark, even if you are sick or on holiday at the time.
- You need to earn £59 or more per week.
- You must write to your employer at least three weeks before you intend to stop work, asking for your SMP. You need to enclose a copy of form MAT B1, which your GP or midwife will give you at the sixth-month mark.

You get
- 90 per cent of your average pay for the first six weeks;
- £54.55 for up to twelve weeks, although you will stop being paid if you go back to work in this time.

You can work up to the last moment if you wish, unless you have a pregnancy-related illness in the last six weeks. If this happens you will start receiving SMP. If your illness is nothing to do with your pregnancy, you can claim statutory sick pay until your maternity leave and SMP start. If your baby is stillborn after twenty-four weeks, you still qualify for SMP.

Maternity Allowance (MA)

This is for working women who do not qualify for SMP, e.g., those who have given up work or changed jobs during their pregnancy. You receive it for eighteen weeks, beginning any time from eleven weeks before your estimated due date.

To qualify

- You need to have worked and paid full-rate National Insurance contributions for at least twenty-six of the sixty-six weeks before the week your baby is due.
- You must fill in form MAI. This is available at antenatal clinics or Social Security offices. Send it in when you are twenty-six weeks' pregnant. If you have MAT B1 from your GP or midwife, send this at the same time or later. It is important to return the MAI form as soon as you have made the twenty-six National Insurance contributions required.
- If in doubt, put in a claim.

You get

- £47.35 per week if you are self-employed, or unemployed in the fifteenth week before the baby is due.
- £54.55 per week if you were employed in the fifteenth week before the baby is due.

Incapacity Benefit

If you have worked but do not qualify for SMP or MA, but have paid full-rate National Insurance contributions in the last three years, you may be entitled to incapacity benefit.

Put in a claim if you have worked at all in the three years prior to pregnancy or birth – you will soon be told if you are not eligible. Make a claim for maternity allowance as close as you can to the twenty-sixth week of pregnancy, sending form MAT B1 with the claim. If you are not entitled to MA, your benefits agency will automatically assess you for incapacity benefit. You will not get incapacity benefit for weeks in which you work.

To qualify
- You must have made three years' worth of National Insurance contributions prior to your pregnancy.

You get
- £46.15 per week, which can be paid from six weeks prior to the birth until two weeks afterwards.

Maternity Payment from the Social Fund

This is a lump sum awarded to help with the cost of buying items for a new baby. It is available to parents claiming income support, family credit or disability working allowance, and also to parents on income support or family credit who adopt a baby under a year old. You can claim it from eleven weeks before your due date and up to three months after the birth.

To receive it
- Fill in form SF100, which is available at your benefits office. Send it back with form MAT B1. If you are claiming after the baby has been born, return form SF100 with a copy of the baby's birth certificate instead.

You get
- £100 per baby. If you have over £500 in savings, payments will be reduced by £1 for every £1 over £500 that you have saved.

Child Benefit

This is available to everyone.

To receive it
- If you are not sent a claim pack, send off the form on the back of the benefits agency leaflet FB8, *Babies and Benefits*, which is available at social security offices. To find the address in the telephone book, look under Benefits Agency. Phone ahead of your visit, as sometimes the benefit agency closest to you might deal with a different area.

You get
- £10.80 per week for your first baby.
- £8.80 per week for subsequent children.

One-Parent Benefit

This is available to certain people bringing up a child on their own. You claim it in the same way as child benefit.

You get
- £6.30 per week.

If you are on income support you may also be entitled to:
- family credit;
- housing benefit;
- council tax benefit;
- health benefits, such as free milk and help with hospital fares.

Free Prescriptions and Dentistry

Prescriptions and dental treatment are free for pregnant women and new mothers who have given birth within the last twelve months (even if the baby died). You should be given a Family Health Services Authority exemption certificate by your doctor. Show this when collecting prescription medicines or receiving dental treatment. Don't forget to tell your dentist you are pregnant before he or she treats you.

State Pensions

If you want to protect your state retirement pension while you are caring for your child at home, ring freeline Social Security on 0800 666 555 and ask about home responsibilities protection (HRP). This reduces the number of years you need to have worked to be entitled to a basic pension, although you will still have to have worked for a minimum of twenty years when you retire to benefit. A woman normally needs thirty-nine qualifying years for a 100 per cent basic pension. If she works for only twenty qualifying years she will receive 52 per cent of her pension but if in addition she has applied for HRP for, say, nineteen years spent at home caring for her children, she will get 75 per cent of her full basic pension.

Financial Planning for You and Your New Baby

A child will cost its parents a minimum of £33,600 before it is sixteen, according to the Legal & General. If you opt for private education, this rises to a knee-weakening £84,000. It is therefore wise to plan your expenditure as far as is possible. It is also important to protect your family by making a will.

Wills

Seven out of ten British people die without making a will. This means that:

- The law decides what happens to your legacy rather than you and your family.
- If you are not married to your partner and one of you dies, the other might have no legal rights to the family home or possessions.

The advantages of making a will
- You decide what happens to your money and possessions.
- It can be used to appoint a legal guardian, someone of your choice, to care for your child in the event of your death.
- Your beneficiaries will receive your bequest relatively quickly. Where there is no legally recognized will it can be many years before the proceeds of the estate are finally handed out.

It is not a good idea to use the DIY will forms available at stationers because in legal terms many different interpretations can be placed upon what may at first appear to be completely straightforward instructions. As a result it may not be possible for your wishes to be carried out in the way you intended.
- Some charities offer free guides to making wills, among them Sight Savers International (tel. 01444 412424) and the British Red Cross (tel. 0171 235 5454 or 201 5044). A free videopack is available from solicitors Leo B. Wallwork & Co. in partnership with UNICEF as part of their home wills service on freephone 0500 223618.

Savings Accounts

Building Society Accounts

Better rates are offered for deposit accounts where thirty or more days' notice of withdrawal has to be given. There are some societies which allow withdrawals to be made without loss of interest if notice has not been given. Similar accounts with the clearing banks do not generally allow instant access without penalties.

> **PLUS POINTS**
> * May put you in good stead should you wish to apply for a mortgage.
> * Very secure form of investment.

For children

To ensure that on your child's account interest will be paid gross and no tax will be deducted, complete form R85, which is available from your local tax office.

National Savings

Available from the Post Office.

> **PLUS POINTS**
> * You have access to your money eight working days after the account is opened with most schemes.
> * Interest is paid in full with no deductions for tax, unlike a building society account.
> * Absolute security of your savings.
> * The network of branches extends to all main and sub-post offices.
> * If you want to open an account in a child's name, you can choose between different schemes, depending on how old you want him to be before he has access to his money.
>
> **MINUS POINTS**
> * Somewhat impersonal service. You cannot expect more than a leaflet or helpline number from counter staff should you need assistance.
> * Withdrawals for larger sums must be made by post.
> * Some index-linked schemes need to be held for five years to be worthwhile.
> * You will get a better rate at certain building societies if you shop around.

For children

National Savings accounts suitable for children include the ordinary account, on which anyone can earn up to £70 a year tax-free, and the investment account, on which interest is taxable but is paid in full. The minimum contribution for the ordinary account is £10 and for the investment account, £20.

National Savings Capital Bonds

For details ask at your post office. For the current interest rate, call 0171 605 9483/4. These are an excellent way of saving, especially when interest rates are high.

PLUS POINTS
* A good rate of interest if the bonds are held for five years.
* Interest is paid gross.

MINUS POINTS
* You must give eight days' notice to withdraw any money.
* The minimum commitment is £100.

National Savings Children's Bonus Bonds

For children under sixteen, these pay tax-free interest (currently 7.85 per cent) if held for five years or more, and a bonus is paid every five years. The bond will be in the child's name but the certificate is sent to the parents or guardians. The minimum investment is £25, and additional bonds must be in multiples of £25, to a maximum of £1,000 (you can buy more than one issue). The child can take control of the fund at sixteen, but there are no further returns beyond the age of twenty-one. According to National Savings, 'There's not a penny due in tax, even if the child becomes a taxpayer in the meantime.'

National Savings-Backed Premium Bonds

These do not generate interest but each month your child has a chance of winning over £1 million or one of a range of lower-value pay-outs. All winnings are tax-free. The initial minimum purchase is £100, and you can add to this, increasing the chances of a win, in multiples of £10.

Premium bonds give better odds than the National Lottery. As prizes are free of tax they are particularly attractive to higher-rate taxpayers. Their computer, 'Ernie', pays out about 5.2 per cent of the total value of bonds in issue as prizes each year.

Children under sixteen cannot buy premium bonds themselves but their parents, grandparents or guardians can purchase them as a gift. For more details ask at your post office.

Tax-Exempt Special Savings Accounts (TESSAs)

TESSAs, a 'no-lose' building society account with competitive rates of interest, are underrated. If you do have to take out your money, you are simply back to square one.

You can invest up to £9,000 over a five-year period and earn a tax-free market rate of interest. Tax is deducted while you save but given back to you at the end. As rates are constantly changing, you are best advised to look at the family finance sections of the weekend press for up-to-date comparisons of the terms offered by different banks and building societies. The better rates are generally given by smaller building societies, which are the most competitive for savers' money.

It is often possible to set up a monthly payment into a TESSA from a current account held at the same bank or building society, which makes the administration painless.

There is now a new scheme enabling investors to carry forward their tax-free savings into a new TESSA fund.

PLUS POINT
* This is a good way of building up tax-free savings.

MINUS POINT
* If capital is withdrawn during the five years, the tax benefits are lost and tax is deducted from the interest paid.

Borrowing

If you need to borrow money to help meet the expenses of a new baby, authorized overdrafts from your bank tend to be cheaper than personal loans. The saving varies – early in 1995, for instance, there was an interest-rate difference between overdrafts and personal loans of 3 per cent at the Halifax, but 10 per cent at the Nationwide. It is also worth approaching your bank or building society to see if they will agree to a 'holiday' period or reduced rate of mortgage repayments.

Plastic is best avoided, but if you do have to resort to it a credit card is often better value than a store card. In December 1995 Burton Group and Debenhams were charging at least 26.30 per cent on their store cards, compared to Mastercards from Save & Prosper and the Royal Bank of Scotland, both of which offered just over 14.5 per cent. Compare rates from different organizations before deciding.

Home Banking

If you are worried about being housebound or don't fancy taking the pram and infant into the bank, consider a telephone banking service, such as Midland's First Direct (tel. 0113 276 6100) and PhoneBank, a TSB service (tel. Freecall 0500 758758).

Equity-Based Investments

Starting a share portfolio is not worthwhile if you have less than £50,000 to invest. To put smaller sums to use on the stockmarket, look at a pooled scheme such as a unit or investment trust. However, you should not consider any of these investments if you have to take out your money after six months because the benefits are only to be seen over five to ten years.

Whereas interest-bearing accounts protect your capital, in equity-based investments it can diminish. However, in the long run, and particularly at times of economic growth, investments that depend on the success and desirability of shares in companies can do rather better than deposits with building societies. The key advice with savings is to spread your money over different types of investments, and this is particularly true with shares, unit and investment trusts.

Unit-trust and investment-trust companies allow you to invest a regular sum each month through their management companies, and indeed this is the cheapest way to acquire an interest in this type of pooled savings. Regular monthly investment has the further benefit of averaging out the cost over the period of the investment, thus making the timing of the investment less critical.

Personal equity plans (PEPs), unit trusts and shares should not be considered as a home for cash that may be needed unexpectedly as their value can fall below the value of the original investment.

Investment is a complicated business, so you should seek professional advice. If you want to save for a specific expense such as school fees, an independent financial adviser can prepare tailor-made investment plans for you.

To whom should I go for advice?

You need an experienced professional you can trust. If you have a good relationship with your accountant, talk to him or her (try to arrange to pay a flat fee in advance of the appointment). Your accountant will probably be more objective than someone whose views may be coloured by the commission he will earn by recommending a particular savings institution. Your accountant should rebate any commission to you or credit it towards other work that he undertakes on your behalf. You should *always* ask for a breakdown of the remuneration received from a plan-provider or investment manager.

Watch out

- Freebies or glossy literature are not good reasons to favour a particular investment.
- A scheme which has 'young' or 'child' in the title does not necessarily offer the best returns.
- If you decide to approach a bank or building society for investment advice, ask if they genuinely can offer a full range of products or whether they are tied to a particular insurance company or can offer only their own schemes.
- An independent financial adviser should be a member of the Personal Investment Authority (PIA), the industry's supervisory body.

Reputable companies offering the full range of products include: Mercury Asset Management, M&G, Henderson Administration and most major merchant banks. PIA tel. 0171 538 8860.

Unit Trusts

Available from financial advisers. Unit trusts involve buying units of a large share portfolio run by a fund manager. The Association of Unit Trusts and Investment Funds (tel. 0171 831 0898) will provide lists of suitable funds and advice and the magazine *Family Finance* is also useful.

PLUS POINTS
* If you want to invest on the stockmarket, the risk is greatly reduced because you are spreading it.
* As a long-term investment, unit trusts can perform extremely well.

MINUS POINT
* High charges can apply, both at the time of purchase (3 to 6 per cent) and in the form of annual management charges, typically between 1 and 1.5 per cent.

Investment Trusts

Another option is the investment trust, available through stockbrokers and financial advisers. These are similar to a unit trust, as they spread risk amongst numerous holdings. Investment trusts are companies which are themselves listed on the Stock Exchange which specialize in buying other companies' shares whose shares can be bought on the Stock Market. Investment trusts are less restricted by rules and regulations than unit trusts. For example, fund managers can borrow various currencies in order to improve profits. Contact the Association of Investment Trust Companies (tel. 0171 588 5347) for details.

Management fees are usually between 1 and 1.5 per cent. You can reduce the costs involved in buying investment trust schemes by investing through a regular savings scheme.

Personal Equity Plans (PEPs)

These are available from virtually all fund managers, many banks and many of the leading building societies. They are usually a good way of saving if you are paying capital gains tax, but otherwise they have little to offer.

> **PLUS POINTS**
> * The government allows each adult to invest up to £6,000 a year in a PEP with tax-free income and gains.
> * There are also a number of hybrid PEPs, such as corporate PEPs, which invest in single companies (and in which you can invest £3,000 more than in a personal PEP) and, most recently, corporate-bond PEPs, for investment in high-yielding debt issued by companies. There is less chance of capital growth with a corporate-bond PEP, but sound prospects of accruing high income in a tax-free environment.
>
> **MINUS POINTS**
> * The administration costs in some cases have been found to outweigh the advantages of tax-free income and capital growth.
> * PEPs can go down as well as up.

Life-Assurance Savings Plans

These can be based on a 'with-profits' insurance policy, which means that, with the right policy, the interest is tax-free once the policy matures (usually after ten years), and because it is 'with profits', the annual bonuses added to the investment cannot be taken away later. There is usually a large terminal bonus, too, paid on maturity. As you are only given a certain yield, you should telephone for a quote or ask an independent financial adviser to research the market on your behalf.

For example, if you were to invest £10,000 with Eagle Star you would receive £17,976 in ten years' time, based on 1995 PIA figures. Improved terms are available for larger amounts.

Alternatively a regular saving of £50 per month would produce £8,950 after ten years, once again based on rates approved by the regulatory body, the PIA.

With an insurance-based savings scheme you can pay for additional life cover so that a lump sum will be paid out for your child in the event of one or both parents' death. You may find it better to have separate policies for your life and your investments.

Tax

Babies and Tax

Until April 1996, a baby's tax allowance is £3,525. Tax must be paid on any income generated from investments or savings in excess of this sum. Parents must pay tax on cash gifts to their offspring, or a baby's bank account that generates more than £100 interest a year, but gifts from other relations or friends are unaffected by this rule. If you fill in form R85 when you open the account, you can receive the interest before tax is deducted (i.e., gross) and pay the tax separately later.

Parents and Tax

Parents have their own tax allowances: an annual capital gains tax exemption of £6,000 each; an income-tax allowance of £3,525 each per year and the married couple's allowance of £1,720 a year. The single parent's allowance is £1,720 in addition to the basic £3,525.

As mothers who stop work to have children rarely use all their personal allowances, tax can be avoided if family savings are put in the mother's name. The Inland Revenue reckons that there are 15 million people – mainly non-working mothers – who are paying unnecessary tax on their savings accounts when they are entitled to receive interest tax-free. Many of these women are also entitled to a refund on the tax they have paid since giving up work, but don't realize that this can be reclaimed.

Make sure that tax is not deducted at source from these investments (you need form R85 again). If in doubt, ask your local tax office for the leaflet 1R110, *A Guide for People with Savings*. This contains two forms: a repayment claim for overpaid tax, and a copy of form R85.

This section was written with the assistance of Barry Stillerman, Personal Finance Partner, of BDO Stoy Hayward, 8 Baker Street, London W1M 1DA, tel. 0171 486 5888, and David Ferman, of Gloucester Place Consultants Limited, 182 Gloucester Place, London NW1 6DS, tel. 0171 723 9382.

PART TWO
PARENTS AS CONSUMERS

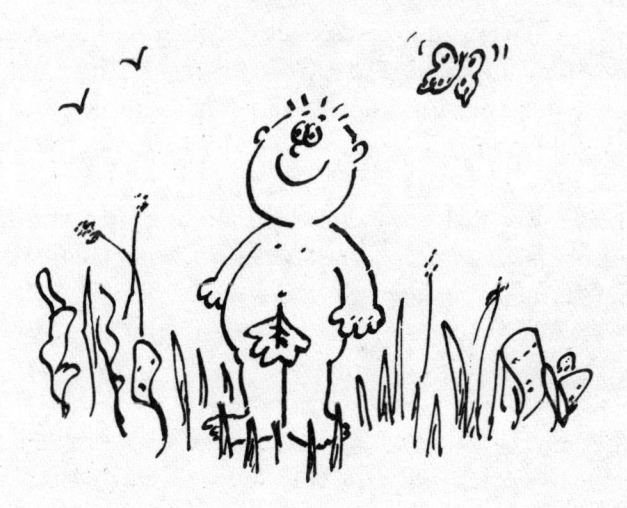

4 Buying and Hiring

Shopping for Your Baby

High Street Stores

Virtually every shop in the high street now claims to be baby-friendly, but some are far more so than others. Free samples for pregnant mothers are offered by Boots, Children's World, Mothercare and Sainsburys. Your clinic or GP should give you claim cards for some of these.

These stores are obvious sources of baby products, but there are others, such as Debenhams, which bend over backwards to assist family shoppers and it would be hard to beat Littlewoods' Index or Argos for good value for nursery equipment and toys.

ASDA

What they sell:
* Baby clothes.
* Food and toiletries.
* Toys and books.

Special services:
* Eighty-two per cent of stores have purpose-built nappy-changing facilities and help is available in all outlets.
* There are twenty-two crèches attached to different stores.
* The ASDA Club Card is currently on trial, offering points towards vouchers and items in a brochure.
* Promotional evenings are arranged locally.
* In some stores, child reins are available.
* Look out for the 'big shopper' checkout with speedy scanners and packers available.

In a national-newspaper survey, ASDA came top in a group of major retailers in terms of good prices and excellent facilities for mothers and babies.

BhS (formerly British Home Stores)

What they sell:
* Baby clothes.
* Nursery lights, bedlinen, throws.
* Embroidered towels for boys and girls.

Special services:
* If there is not a lift available you can use the staff lift if you are accompanied by a member of staff.
* Mother-and-baby changing rooms.
* Customer-card save-as-you-spend scheme called Choice, which offers up to 15 per cent off merchandise for up to a year. Special evenings are arranged for Choice customers.

Boots

What they sell:
The larger branches sell a superb range of products for new mothers:
* Maternity underwear.
* Nursery decoration.
* Safety gadgets.
* Baby food.
* Feeding equipment.
* Baby and children's clothing.
* Toiletries and medicines for mothers and babies.

Special services:
* Baby-and-child advisers and baby consultants in larger stores.
* Promotional evenings for expectant mothers in certain stores.
* Free nappy-delivery service.
* TENS hire in larger stores (see Chapter 7).
* Baby-changing facilities in larger stores.

Boots has maintained the traditional values of offering quality products sold by well-trained staff. It is the only high-street store which can offer baby-and-child advisers (trained nurses or midwives) and baby consultants. Look in the back of their Baby & Child catalogue to see which branches employ these paragons. It is worth getting to know your local baby adviser/consultant, who will give you information about all the baby products Boots sell, other pregnancy products and help you select the items most suited to your needs. The consultants also make a real effort to build relationships with local families. Boots are very conscious of their chemist's background and extremely careful in researching and developing their own-brand products. The Mother's Recipe baby-food line, which is fully organic, features some excellent meals. The Baby & Child catalogue, which has a number of useful discount vouchers in the back, is on sale in all stores, price 50p.

Useful free leaflets (again, with discount vouchers) can be found around the store. The current *Breastfeeding* leaflet includes a £2 voucher valid when you spend £10 or more on any breastfeeding products. For visually impaired people, there is a catalogue of Christmas gifts prepared each year on tape and in Braille. Your local store should have details.

Children's World

What they sell:
* A huge range of baby equipment and safety gadgets.
* Baby food.
* Baby clothes, including a premature baby range.
* Toys.
* Toiletries.

Special services:
* Special order facility for parents with particular requirements.
* Free 'MOT' for pushchairs and buggies.
* Play area, children's hairdresser and children's shoe shops in larger branches.

At the time of writing Children's World is part of Boots, so you can buy Boots' own-brand products there, among others. There is plenty of parking, so if you want to buy a car seat you can try it out in your car before you buy it. Staff are trained to specialize in certain product areas, so if you want expert advice, go on a weekday when they are more likely to be able to spend time with you. Ask about seasonal discounts on large purchases. Good access makes Children's World stores particularly useful for disabled customers. But this may change if the proposed takeover by Storehouse, owners of Mothercare, goes through.

Debenhams

What they sell:
* Baby clothes.
* Nursery furniture.
* Toiletries.
* Toys.

Special services:
* Changing facilities in all stores.
* Lifts and escalators.
* Debenhams' account card, which offers 10 per cent off sales during your first week, customer account evenings/previews, notice of sales and other helpful information.
* Delivery service for all local customers.
* Collect-by-car facilities.
* Restaurants have highchairs, a children's menu, bottle-warming service, assistance with trays and a play area if space permits.

An increasing number of Debenhams stores offer a 'World of Brighter Futures', a haven for desperate parents with older children in tow on a wet Saturday. This is a floor with a theme-park atmosphere dedicated to children. Computers, records, toys, games, clothes (from 0 to 14 years) and nursery decorations are well laid out and sold by seemingly saint-like staff. 'We encourage the kids to play with all the toys,' said one manager. 'We don't mind all the mess – we want them to have fun.'

Early Learning Centre

What they sell:
At larger stores:
* A full range of baby equipment, available by mail order.
* Nursery decorations including wallpaper, fabrics.
* Toys.

Special services:
* Home delivery for larger items.
* A new mail-order catalogue twice a year.
* Larger stores have nappy-changing facilities and a toilet. In smaller branches, the staff will always find you somewhere to change your baby.

The Early Learning Centre's nursery department is so good that it is not unknown for people to come in and buy entire window displays. They do a small, upmarket range which features co-ordinates from duvets and wallpapers in the bedroom down to the last flannel in the bathroom. They also have a selection of good-quality equipment: buggies, highchairs etc., and a fun range of baby and children's clothes. New openings of larger ELCs are scheduled – keep an eye on the local press for details.

Littlewoods

What they sell:
* Baby clothes.
* Baggy tops.
* Index, the catalogue shop within Littlewoods, offers good-value cots, toys and buggies.

Special services:
* Parent-and-baby rooms available in stores with restaurants.
* Promotional evenings and a customer card may be available in the future.
* Home delivery for Index customers.
* Will refund the difference if you find the same product cheaper elsewhere.

John Lewis

What they sell:
* Childrenswear (except at High Wycombe Furnishing & Leisure).
* Baby-equipment range depends on size of store, but generally includes prams, cots, mattresses and feeding systems.
* Nursery decorations, soft furnishings and fabrics.
* Toiletries.
* Nappies.
* Maternity wear and underwear (except at High Wycombe).
* Lighting and electrical goods.
* Towels.

Special services:
* Baby-changing facilities are available in all stores. You will need to ask in smaller outlets.
* Good access to all floors.
* Free delivery is within a thirty-mile radius of the store. Customer collection points allow shoppers to pick up their goods by car.
* Parents with children are encouraged to ask staff for help.

John Lewis is *the* place for mummies buying equipment for their pregnant daughters. Their own brand, Jonelle, is top quality and competitively priced. The department store with the 'Never knowingly undersold' slogan can be a casualty of its own popularity, so if an extremely long order time is quoted, ring around smaller shops in your area to see if they can get the product in faster.

If Mummy has already announced her intention to kit you out at John Lewis, it is essential to go at a reasonably quiet time – it is no fun standing in queues when you are pregnant. If the assistant's knowledge seems suspect, find another member of staff who knows his or her stuff. When they are good, they are very, very good, and help you to steer clear of unsuitable products.

Marks & Spencer

What they sell:
* Bras. Trained fitters are available in larger stores.
* Baggy tops.
* Nursery furniture and decorations (in larger stores).
* Prepared vegetables for cooking and puréeing for baby food.
* Baby clothes.
* Toiletries.

Special services:
* Mail order.
* Lifts in modern stores.
* Delivery/collect-by-car service (larger stores).
* Flower-delivery service.
* If you ask for assistance at the till, someone will come and help you to pack your bags.

Although you may find only a few items at smaller stores, the larger outlets have beautifully co-ordinated ranges of baby clothes. Buy while you see: the more popular lines tend to disappear within hours. If you need a present for someone else's baby and do not know the sex, there are plenty of white items.

Mothercare

What they sell:
Virtually everything you can think of for pregnancy and birth.
* Maternity wear and underwear.
* Nursery furniture and decorations.
* Safety gadgets.
* Prams and buggies.
* Feeding equipment.
* Baby and children's wear.
* Toiletries for mother and baby.

Special services:
* Lifts or escalators in newer stores.
* Delivery/collect-by-car service.
* Extensive mail-order catalogue.

Dynamic young buyers are transforming Mothercare's merchandise and their products are now both delightful and practical. The company imposes stringent conditions on its suppliers to ensure that only quality products are sold. They also guarantee their pushchairs for twelve months. To get the best out of your local branch, try to go in on a quieter shopping day. Staff specialize in certain areas of stock, so if you want a buggy, check that you are talking to the 'buggy expert' before you buy.

An extensive *First Baby Guide* (50p in all stores) allows you to order everything you could possibly want for your new baby without the hassle of going into town, and most items can be delivered within seven working days. But if you have the time there is no substitute for going and testing the goods in the shop. Mothercare stocks plenty of products in addition to those featured in the *First Baby Guide*.

Safeway

What they sell:
* Baby food.
* Baby clothing (selected stores).
* Nappies.
* Toiletries.

Special services:
* Customer Connections scheme – evening meetings with Safeway directors for customers to suggest improvements.
* Family Connections – a panel of 1,500 parents to test new products and facilities.
* Parent-and-baby rooms in 50 per cent of stores. Fathers are welcome to use the facilities if nursing mothers are not embarrassed.
* Bag-packing and carry-out service.
* Fresh flower-delivery.
* Six different types of shopping trolley for babies and children.
* Nineteen stores have crèches run by qualified nursery nurses.
* ABC customer card. One point given for every £1 spent, which can be redeemed against a range of products and services, including family days out and money off shopping.

Sainsbury

What they sell:
* Baby food.
* Toiletries.
* Own-brand nappies.
* Toys and books.

Special services:
* Changing facilities in most stores, especially new and larger ones. A room is always made available where a purpose-built facility does not exist.
* Free Sainsbury Performers nappies available in most baby-changing rooms.
* Baby food and milk-warming in coffee shops.
* Baby welcome pack.
* Loyalty cards in two-thirds of stores.
* Parent-and-child parking available in 225 store car parks.
* Child-sized trolleys available in addition to the ten different types for elderly and disabled customers and those shopping with children.
* If you cannot find a product, a shop assistant will take you to it rather than just give you directions.
* Packers available at peak times.
* If you get to the checkout and realize that you have forgotten something, a member of staff will fetch it for you.
* Assistants will carry shopping to your car on request.

Sainsbury have won numerous plaudits for their helpfulness. Their own-brand make-up is one of the best and cheapest ways to give yourself a new look during pregnancy, and magazines' beauty editors seem to favour the bronzer in particular.

If you have a sudden burst of energy and affluence, Sainsbury's Savacentres stock not only baby clothes but a huge variety of tempting products to enhance your household.

> **Tesco**
>
> *What they sell:*
> * Baby clothes.
> * Toiletries.
> * Nappies.
> * Baby food.
>
> *Special services:*
> * Changing facilities in all new stores and a programme of refitting in older ones.
> * Bottle-warming in coffee shops.
> * Nearly all stores are on one floor with automatic doors.
> * The Tesco Clubcard gives you points and discount vouchers when you spend over £10.
> * Parent-and-child parking facilities.
> * A selection of trolleys for carrying children and babies.
> * Flower- and wine-delivery service.

Tesco was voted the UK's most parent-friendly supermarket in the 1994 and 1995 Tommy's Campaign Awards. It was also Retailer of the Year in the 1994 Mother & Baby Awards for its facilities for pregnant women and people with young children.

Their skincare range is worth experimenting with if you find pregnancy is causing problems you do not usually experience.

> **Woolworth**
>
> *What they sell:*
> * Baby clothes.
> * Toiletries.
> * Toys.
>
> *Special services:*
> * Changing facilities in branches with cafés.
> * Help is always available on request.

If you want to know more about shoppers' rights, debit card company Visa Delta has produced *The Visa Delta Shopping Handbook*. For a free copy call 0171 231 5432.

Waitrose

What they sell:
* Baby food.
* Nappies.
* Toiletries.

Special services:
* All shops with toilets (which include toilets for disabled customers) include baby-changing facilities. Where there are no customer toilets assistants will be happy to escort parents and children to use Waitrose staff facilities.
* Shopping is all on one level.
* The Waitrose account card offers up to fifty-six days' interest-free credit and the lowest monthly interest rate in the country.
* Mail-order flowers with chocolates and wine. Freephone 0800 592761 to order flowers before 2 p.m. for next-day delivery. Telephone 0181 543 0966 for details of wine deliveries.
* Gift vouchers can be used in both Waitrose and John Lewis stores.
* A range of trolleys incorporates different-sized children's seats.
* Parent-and-child parking bays are being introduced.
* Party-food service, including sandwiches, christening and birthday cakes.

Independent Retailers

Products in this book are usually mentioned in the context of larger chain stores such as Mothercare simply to ensure that people all over Britain have access to the goods discussed – if not in the high street, by mail order. This does not mean you should ignore your local independent retailer. Nursery equipment shops tend to be excellent – especially if they are in a town that also supports large chain stores. They have to be able to offer good prices and a first-class service in order to stay in business. Some of them have built up relationships with particular suppliers that allow them to offer large discounts. Telephone Bounty on 01733 361361 for details of independents near you.

We were particularly impressed by the following:

Babycare, 34 Burleigh Street, Cambridge CB 1DG, tel. 01223 355296.
Babycentre, Mam House, Roseville Road, Leeds LS8 5RQ, tel. 01132 428473.
Diddyland, 24 Goose Gate, Nottingham, tel. 0115 9580731.
Glasgow Pram Centre, 76 Gallowgate, Glasgow, tel. 0141 552 3998.
Lilliput, 278 Upper Richmond Road, London SW15 6TQ, tel. 0181 780 1682 (will deliver anywhere in the world).
The Baby's Room, 11 Tunsgate, Guildford GU1 3QT, tel. 01483 578984.
Nippers, a chain of franchises based in converted barns on farms. Prices tend to be low because they have none of the overheads suffered by inner city retailers and they have negotiated good deals with a range of suppliers. If you live in the country or are going for a rural day out, telephone: 01732 838333/838334/832243 to see if there is a branch nearby. Your family can enjoy the farm animals while you burn a hole in your chequebook. Parking is no problem – a particular benefit if you want to buy a car seat. Saturdays may be exceptionally busy.

There are specialist outlets that sell equipment designed for twins and multiples. See pages 42–4, 283–4 and 341.

Help us to make *The Baby Bible* better
If you have found any excellent products or services that are not mentioned, please get in touch and let us know. Information should go to Mr D. Reed, Baby Bible, 172 Greenford Road, Harrow, Middlesex HA1 3QZ.

Equipment Hire

Before you buy any major pieces of equipment, you might consider hiring. It is a good way to test the various options and it offers an immediate solution to parents whose babies arrive early. Most equipment hire is for families holidaying abroad, but if you are travelling in Britain, you can arrange equipment hire near your destination so that you do not have to waste vast amounts of car space on baby paraphernalia.

The Babyline, on 01831 310355, will give you the telephone number of the nearest member of the British Equipment Hirers Association. Otherwise people in the Leeds area should call 0113 278 5560 direct. Many independent nursery-equipment shops hire out a range of items at competitive rates.

Average Costs for Hiring Baby Equipment

Item	1 week	2 weeks	1 month	3 months
Cots				
Small travel cot	£ 8.60	£13.20	£18.90	£28.40
Large travel cot	£10.00	£15.60	£21.80	£33.40
Buggies				
Basic	£ 7.60	£12.00	£16.40	£22.60
Reclining	£ 9.10	£14.40	£19.50	£28.70
Twin basic	£10.60	£15.40	£22.10	£30.80
Tandem	£12.70	£18.80	£26.20	£40.90
Car seats				
Baby carriers	£ 6.60	£10.00	£13.10	£17.00
Other types	£ 8.00	£13.00	£17.80	£25.30
Miscellaneous				
Highchairs	£ 7.90	£12.10	£16.10	£23.80
Baby diners	£ 5.80	£ 7.80	£10.80	£14.70
Backpacks	£ 6.90	£10.70	£14.60	£20.60
Bouncers	£ 5.10	£ 7.40	£10.50	£15.30
Baby walkers	£ 6.00	£ 9.00	£11.30	£16.60
Stair gates	£ 5.10	£ 7.20	£ 9.70	£13.50
Fireguards	£ 5.20	£ 7.40	£10.10	£13.20

Source: BEHA survey conducted in 1995.

Bleep hire

To keep in contact with your partner nearing labour time, you can hire a parent pager from London Pager (tel. 0800 592383).

The minimum hire period is twelve weeks (£55 plus a £50 refundable deposit). They also offer a one-year hire. Pager Rentals (tel. 01733 319454) will supply a pager for a shorter period. Two weeks' hire is £16, three weeks £21, and four weeks £24.

British Standards

Over sixty standards govern the manufacture of nursery products. Children can inflict terrible damage on anything they come into contact with: toys, feeding dishes, transport, siblings – they don't distinguish between what is meant to be bashed around and dismantled and what isn't. More importantly, manufacturers must ensure that as well as being babyproof, nursery products cannot harm the child.

The standards for nursery equipment all demand a level of general safety in terms of finger traps, limb traps and toxicity of materials. They also deal with more specific areas of risk related to individual pieces of equipment. Nigel Overton at BSI Product Certification says, 'The Kitemark can say volumes more about the safety of a product than a good shake on the shop floor ever could.'

Pushchairs

The British standards dictate that a pushchair has a minimum of two locking devices. The main lock can be manual or automatic, but the safety lock must be automatic. In addition, pushchairs mustn't crumple like a boneless crinoline when they bump into a kerb.

Even the most doting parents are unlikely to wheel their offspring non-stop from Manchester to Fort William, but if their pushchair has been tested at BSI, it will have been subjected to an equivalent journey. Test engineers tether pushchairs to a rig called a rolling road, a lumpy metal conveyor belt, for a continuous sixty-four-hour, 320-kilometre trek. The pushchair is then tested for rigidity, stability and braking or locking efficiency. The engineers place the pushchair on a slope to check its parking mechanisms and its stability, and use 15kg metal cylinder test dummies to ensure that it won't tip over when in use.

Nursery Furniture

Stability tests are a common feature in many standards relating to childcare articles. Children are unstable items: they rock back and forth and lean over the sides of whatever they're sitting in as they try to grab whatever it is that's just out of reach. To make sure that the highchair, cot or playpen and the child stay upright, an impact test, using a device similar to a swinging demolition ball, smacks into the equipment to check that it won't topple over or fall apart.

The standard for playpens, BS4863, takes account of children's tendency to sink their teeth into anything they can fit into their mouths. It specifies that a child should not be able to bite through the padding around the rim of the pen. Laboratory engineers use an instrument that looks like a small chisel head, which is designed to imitate the properties of a child's tooth. They apply this to the padding with a force of 60 Newtons. The material should stay intact and the foam inside the rim should remain inaccessible to the child.

Europe

The European standard BSI represents the UK on European committees and will gradually replace the British standard, but BSI will continue to test products. 'What we think is safe and what the other nationalities think is safe are often worlds apart,' says Peter Jackson, technical director at Maclaren. For instance, most parents in Britain would no more put their child into an unharnessed highchair than they would drive without a seatbelt. In Germany, however, parents feel it is psychologically damaging to restrain a child, while the Norwegians would rather risk a child falling out of a highchair or buggy than expose them to what they see as a risk of strangulation.

The above is adapted from an article in BSI News.

The Baby Products Association

The Baby Products Association aims to promote the baby and nursery products industry to both the general public and the trade. It represents the industry to government departments in the UK, EC and elsewhere, as well as to local authorities and other organizations with an interest in this field. It is heavily involved in the development of British and European standards and operates a code of practice for the sale and repair of wheeled goods. For a copy of the code, please send an SAE to the Baby Products Association, Erlegh Manor, Vicarage Road, Pitstone, Leighton Buzzard, Bedfordshire LU7 9EY.

5   Safety

Avoiding Accidents

Nearly eight hundred thousand British children under five visit hospital each year as a result of an accident. Seventy-five children die and two thousand are injured in house fires. Fifty thousand under-fives go to hospital after falling downstairs, and forty-five thousand with suspected poisoning (Child Accident Prevention Trust figures).

You can do a lot to keep your baby out of harm's way by storing household products and medicines out of reach and fitting safety equipment. Many people start to think about alarms, gates and child locks around the time their baby is born. Children develop quickly and your home must be ready to cope with their new enthusiasms.

> !!! One of the best aids to safety is a telephone-answering machine or a portable handset. Many an accident has been caused by a parent rushing for the phone.

First-Aid Information

The St John Ambulance Brigade has produced a video called *Breath of Life*, which shows you how to administer artificial ventilation and chest compression to a baby or young child. It is available by mail order from St John Ambulance (tel. 0171 278 7888) at £10.95 plus £3.50 postage and packing. They also supply another video, *In Safe Hands*, which covers extensive first aid. The cost is £9.99 plus postage and packing. You might like to club together with the other members of your antenatal classes and share the cost.

The St John Ambulance also runs Lifesaver for Babies and Children courses in which parents can practise techniques under instruction. The price is approximately £15 to £25 – it varies from county to county – for the four-hour course. For further details, contact your local St John Ambulance – the telephone number will be in the phone book – or their central office on 0171 235 5231.

> !!! You should keep a first-aid kit in your home and car.

Around the Home

Home Safety Assessments

Many health visitors will be glad to look round your home to identify potential danger areas and advise on how to correct them. If you don't already have a health visitor, contact your GP.

Kiddiproof produce a home safety starter pack (price £12) which contains socket covers, a fridge lock, cupboard and draw catches, easy-to-fit corner cushions for sharp corners on tables and shelves, and a nightlight which slots into a 13-amp socket. Telephone 01243 864404 to place your order.

Doors

If you do not have toughened safety glass, use plastic film over glass doors to prevent a broken pane from splintering. Safety film is available in a 73 × 180cm roll from Mothercare, price

£14.99, including all you need to fit it. If you buy the film elsewhere, check that the pack contains the materials to fix it in place.

If you are installing safety glass ensure that it carries the Kitemark or BS6206.

If your baby suddenly develops a fascination with the cat flap, you may have to consider sealing it for a while.

Prevent doors from slamming and trapping little fingers by fitting a slam protector. Slam Proof from Romkins (£4.99 for a pack of two) ensures that external doors close slowly. For stockists telephone 0161 962 4206. Safety Grip from Brainstorm (£3.99 for two) is a curved piece of foam which slots on to internal doors.

Flooring

You do not want to trip while carrying your baby, especially at the top of the stairs. Make sure that the carpets and rugs are firmly fixed to the floor – a hole or turned-up edge could send you flying. Rug-hold underlay, a non-slip underlay for securing rugs to carpets and carpets to floors, is available at £8.50 per square metre from the John Lewis Carpet Department (tel. 0171 629 7711).

Gates and Barriers for Stairs

All safety gates and barriers must be firmly secured to the wall. You can usually buy extra holding brackets or cups so that you can move the gate to different positions. To be absolutely safe, go for a gate that needs holes drilled in the wall to fix it in place. Those you can remove as and when you need to can give way and cause accidents.

Barriers are cheaper than gates, but not as convenient because they do not open out. Gates open either across the full width of the staircase or in the centre. The ones with a central opening have a bar at the bottom that may cause you to trip if you are not concentrating. Make sure that this section is wide enough to allow you to pass through comfortably. Check what width of gate or barrier you need before buying (if you do make a mistake, extensions are usually available). Gates should conform to BS4125.

Teach your child to come downstairs backwards on his tummy.

Remember that a toddler might attempt to mimic barrier-vaulting if he sees you doing it.

Fitting gates

- Fixing a gate securely is a two-person job.
- If you want to prevent your baby from crawling up the stairs as well as from falling down them, fit gates at both ends of the staircase.
- Where possible, fit your gate on the landing rather than across the top of the stairs. If you step over the gate, it is much safer and easier to do it on a level surface than down on to a stair.
- Board up banisters if there is a chance that a crawler or toddler might slip through them.

★★★ Star buys ★★★

The Bettacare Child Safe Opening Gate (between £24.99 and £27), which closes behind you (tel. 01293 851896).

The Mothercare Wooden Baby Gate (£24.99), does not have a bar at the bottom.

The Tomy Adjust-Width Gate adjusts to fit openings of 69cm to 94cm (£21.99 from the Early Learning Centre).

Smoke Detectors

The four major causes of domestic fires are cooking appliances, cigarettes and matches, heaters and open fires and electrical wiring.

You should have one smoke detector per floor. Look for the

Kitemark or BS5446. Electrical stores will be able to sell you a mains smoke alarm with a back-up battery. Although these are more expensive (about £20) and need to be connected to the mains, they will not require new batteries each year – a battery-operated smoke alarm is only as good as the battery inside it. For large houses, you can buy an interconnected alarm system whereby when one detector senses smoke, they all go off.

Check that the detector:

- is easy to test (First Alert have models you can test with a torch to save having to reach for a button at ceiling level);
- warns you when the battery is low;
- has an integral escape light – fires often knock out lighting round the house.

Gas detectors

If you have an appliance burning gas, coal, oil or solid fuel which is faulty or badly installed, you could be at risk from carbon-monoxide poisoning. The gas is invisible but lethal. A pack of two sticker detectors which you can take on holiday or use at home is available direct from Do It All for £5.99 (including postage and packing). Call 01904 672999 for details.

Kitchen

When you are buying cleaning fluids, go for the ones with the most childproof lids.

Any potentially dangerous equipment, such as knives, or household materials such as cleaning fluids should be securely shut away. Where you have two cupboard handles close together, you can link them with a thick elastic band to prevent a small toddler from opening them. Buy drawer and cupboard safety catches (around £3.99 for a pack of five) from Boots or Mothercare.

Dissuade your baby from propping himself up on an open dishwasher to inspect the sharp knives and glasses inside. Try to train yourself to load cutlery upside down so that the blades are not sticking upwards.

Every home should have a multi-purpose powder fire extinguisher. If you do a lot of frying, it is a good idea to have a fire blanket close to hand. Do It All sell a fire extinguisher for £19.99.

If your freezer or fridge is at floor level, you can fit freezer locks, such as the Boots Fridge-Freezer Lock £1.99).

A safety guard for your hob, such as the Mothercare hob protector (£14.99), will prevent little hands from pulling down saucepans. A hob guard is four-sided and fits most hobs set into worktops; a cooker guard is three-sided and suits most electric or gas cookers with a back panel. The problem with cooker guards is that it can be tricky to fit pans on to all four rings at the same time.

If you are buying a new hob, do not choose an 'island' model accessible from all four sides as there is nowhere to push heavy, hot pans out of harm's way.

Kettle guards fit most kettles but are rather cumbersome. If you have to buy a new kettle, get a cordless one. You can shorten the cord connection to the base so that it only just reaches the socket. Boil only the amount of water you need: water from the kettle can scald up to fifteen minutes after it has been boiled. Avoid having a hot drink when you have a baby on your lap or close by, in case you are jogged.

Flexes can dangle within a baby's reach.

★★★ Star buy ★★★

Curly flexes that conform to BS6500 are available at £6.50 from Children's World.

Oven doors can get very hot and will retain their heat for some time. You can buy oven guards, but some are difficult to fit and some are opaque, which prevents you from seeing what is in the oven.

★★★ **Star buy** ★★★
Toys R Us Safety First-Brand oven guard (£12.99).

Keep the rubbish bin in a cupboard so that it is not available for inspection, and remember that yanking a tablecloth may seem a good idea to a tiny child.

New washing-machines are often fitted with child locks. If yours does not have one, buy a lock if you think there is any danger of your child loading his toys or even himself into the machine. Boots sell a multi-purpose lock at £2.50.

Bathroom

If you have a bolt on your bathroom door, make sure that it is high up – at adult eye-level – to stop a small child locking himself in.

Bath supports made of plastic, sponge or flannel are designed to keep a baby's head out of direct contact with the bathwater. You should never leave a baby unattended in one of these. A non-slip bath mat is a good idea. Tomy Soft Spout (£2.75) is an inflatable cover which fits over taps to avoid bumped heads or burns from the hot tap.

Fit glass shower screens with safety glass or safety film (see Doors).

If your baby seems fascinated by the toilet, you can buy a lock to keep the seat down.

(See also Bathtime, page 197.)

★★★ **Star buy** ★★★
Boots multi-purpose lock (£2.50).

Bedrooms

If you are concerned that you will not be able to hear your baby if he cries, buy a monitor (see Chapter 13).

If you use a Moses basket or carrycot, never leave it on a chest of drawers or other raised surface when the baby is in it.

Do not place the cot near curtains or a roller-blind cord – your baby might be tempted to pull them or try to swing from them. Cot activity centres should be removed once a child can sit up as he might use them as steps if he decides to climb out.

Low-energy bulbs are a good idea for children's bedrooms because they are cool to the touch. They are designed to last up to eight times longer than a standard bulb and cut electricity costs by over 75 per cent. They are also a good choice for nightlights and hall lights. A 14-watt low-energy bulb is equivalent to a 60-watt conventional bulb and costs around £10. Low-energy bulbs are often available on special offer as manufacturers are keen to promote their use.

Windows

The Bettacare multi-purpose gate, which can be used as a safety gate when a baby is first mobile, doubles as a window barrier. There are two sizes: 62 to 109cm (£24.99) and 108 to 156cm (£29.99). Both are adjustable.

Never open sash windows from the bottom upwards.

Buy window safety catches such as Boots' window lock at £3.99.

If you fit security locks, keep the key on a hook nearby in case of fire. Double-glazed windows can be installed with childproof locks if you ask for them when they are fitted.

Do not put furniture below the window as it may encourage your child to climb on to it.

Drawing Room

If you are concerned that your baby might hit his head on the corner of your coffee table, buy corner protectors such as Boots' corner cushions (£1.75 for four).

Fit a fireguard and fix it to the wall so that your baby cannot pull it over. The Hago fireguard, at £19.50 from most major nursery retailers, is a good one.

If your baby likes 'posting' objects into your video, you can buy a video guard, known in the trade as 'jam sandwich guards'. You will soon discover why . . . The Boots video lock (£1.99) fits most front-loading VHS video-recorders.

Electricity

- Get your wiring checked if it is over fifteen years old.
- Fit plug and socket guards.
- Check that old flexes are not worn or frayed along the length or around the plug. A child may be tempted to suck or chew protruding wires.
- Consider buying residual-current detectors which cut off the power if there is a fault. These are fitted like normal sockets. An RCD socket such as PowerBreaker (£33 for a single and £45 for a double) can be used at high-risk points.

Toys

Buy toys from reputable retailers. Look for the CE mark, the European standard; or BS5665; or the Lion mark of the British Toy and Hobby Association. See Chapter 18 for information on toy safety. There is also a new symbol – a white circle depicting a 'baby face' dissected by a red line and an age, to indicate safety level.

If you are buying garden toys:
- Make sure your sandpit has a lid. It will keep the sand clean.
- Do not get equipment that is too big for the garden.

The DTI Consumer Safety Unit (0171 215 1770) produces a useful free leaflet 'Be Safe With Huggy', which gives safety information in a way that will help parents explain it to older children.

Babies and Other Animals

If you are pregnant or have small children and own a cat or a dog, domestic hygiene is essential. Never let your pet lick the baby's face.

According to the *Independent on Sunday*'s 'Dirty Dogs' campaign, and the Tidy Britain Group, Britain currently produces a thousand tons of dog faeces a day, and with them a spate of scare stories concerning their effects on pregnant women and babies. The medical profession generally advise as follows.

Dogs

Many people find it difficult to reconcile the needs of a pet with the demands of a new baby. Although cats tend to look after themselves, if you are planning to get a dog, think about the following.

- Will you have the time or energy to take a dog out for its daily exercise?
- If the dog is ill, will you be able to take it to the vet and nurse it at home?
- Is the dog house-trained?
- Can you keep it in a separate room from the baby?

Toxocara Canis

This is an extremely rare disease caused by swallowing roundworm eggs, present in some dog faeces. Tiny children are most likely to catch this by accidentally swallowing contaminated soil. Since 1983, there have been two cases of children being blinded in one eye as a result. Call the Pet Health Council Helpline on 01476 861379 for further information.

If you have a dog and small children:
- Keep your dog wormed. Toxocara is destroyed by worming.
- Your child should wash his hands after touching animals and before eating.

- Dispose of your dog's faeces rather than letting your child accidentally land in them in the garden.

Cats

Toxoplasmosis

Toxoplasmosis is an infection transmitted by cat faeces and undercooked meat. It is an exceptionally complex subject and cannot be dealt with in detail here. Although it has little lasting effect on most healthy adults and children, if you catch it when you are pregnant the germ could be transmitted to your baby, who could be born with a congenital birth defect such as blindness or deafness. Miscarriage or stillbirth can also result. The Symptoms are similar to those of 'flu. If you are concerned, consult your GP immediately and ask for a blood test to detect toxoplasmosis antibodies. This should be free of charge. You can avoid the risk of toxoplasmosis by sticking to these rules:

- Wear gloves while gardening, even if you don't own a cat. Someone else's may have wandered into your garden.
- After cooking with raw meat, fresh fruit and vegetables, wash your hands and all kitchen implements and surfaces.
- Don't eat underdone meat.
- If you have to clean out the cat litter, wear rubber gloves. Toxoplasma eggs become infective twenty-four hours after they have left the cat, so the tray should be emptied as soon as the cat has used it and thoroughly cleaned and scalded with boiling water to minimize any risk.
- If you stroke your cat, wash your hands afterwards.

> !!! If you're tempted to cuddle a newborn lamb – don't. Lambing ewes and their offspring lambs can carry ovine chlamydiosis and listeriosis, which can cause severe illness in pregnant women resulting in miscarriage.

Further advice

- Protect your sleeping baby from roaming pets with a pram net (£4 buggy size; £8 cot size); available from NCT Sales, tel. 0141 633 5552.

The RSPCA says:

- If you have to have a cat or a dog, make sure it is small and needs minimal upkeep.
- Don't buy a Rottweiler, pit-bull terrier, Dobermann or any other fighting or guarding dog.
- Don't buy terrapins. They can carry salmonella and need a lot of attention.
- Buy a goldfish, a rabbit or a guinea pig, but keep it well away from your baby.

Helpful organizations

- **The Pet Health Council**, Thistledown Cottage, 49 Main Street, Sewestern, Grantham, Lincs NG33 5RF, tel. 01476 861379, will respond to inquiries on pet health and welfare issues, including worming.
- The **RSPCA**, Causeway, Horsham, West Sussex RH12 1HG, tel. 01403 264181, can offer information on various pet-related subjects.
- The **Toxoplasmosis Trust**, 61–71 Collier Street, London N1 9BE, tel. 0171 713 0663; Helpline 0171 713 0599.
- **Community Hygiene Concern**, 160 Inderwick Road, London N8 9JT, tel. 0181 341 7167, offers information on toxoplasmosis, toxocara canis, and also on parasites such as head lice and threadworm.

6 The Green Parent

Pregnancy and the Environment

Expectant mothers are more likely to care about the environment than any other single group in society. For many women, and men too, the prospect of becoming a parent may make them think deeply about the environment for the first time. As pregnant women and children are more susceptible and vulnerable to illnesses caused by environmental pollution, they might be right to be more concerned.

There is much you can do to lower the pollution levels in your own body before and during pregnancy, and, of course, after you have given birth. Consider the health of both you and your partner before conceiving. If you have had difficulties in getting pregnant you might like to check your pollution levels. Recent scientific reports link organochlorine pollution with infertility. Contact **Foresight**, the association for the promotion of preconceptual care, at 28 The Paddock, Godalming, Surrey GU7 1XD, tel. 01483 427 839.

Avoid toxins and toxic chemicals wherever possible. Cadmium, lead and mercury are found in batteries and in pesticides used on foods. Cleaning products can contain chlorine bleach, phosphates, sodium perborate, formaldehyde and sulphuric acid. These can not only be irritating and make you nauseous, they can also be deadly. Clear your house of chemical pollution and try to reduce the risk of inhaling chemicals which can destroy some of the essential trace elements so important for a healthy foetus. For instance, lead pollution can lower the amount of manganese and zinc in the body – both chemicals which are crucial for healthy sperm and pregnancy.

Avoid disinfectants. Perhaps from a misplaced desire to keep everything exceptionally clean, we can unwittingly damage our environment and our own health. According to Karen Christensen in *Home Ecology* (Arlington Books) a large number of disinfectants contain cresol, a chemical which can affect the central nervous system and cause organ damage. There are alternatives which have not been tested on animals, such as the Caurnie Soaperie's DES disinfectant, which can be found in good health-food stores. (Call 0141 776 1218 for stockists.)

Your Diet

Research indicates that your prenatal nutritional condition is the most important factor in influencing a good pregnancy and a healthy baby. To lower your own pollution intake and ensure the best possible environment for your child, eat organic food wherever possible. Studies suggest that organic food has more absorbable vitamins and minerals than other foods, and obviously it has no chemical additions. Most good supermarkets sell organic food and will do their best to stock it if you ask. Inquire locally about organic-box schemes whereby food is delivered to your door for a fixed price.

The **Soil Association**, 86–88 Colston Street, Bristol, Avon BS1 5BB, tel. 01179 290661, will give information on the standards and availability of organic foods, and supply a *Go Organic* regional guide.

Organic-box schemes

Organic Direct, Liverpool, tel. 0151 734 1919. Fruit and vegetables, cereal products, dried fruits and seeds.

Organic Roundabout, Birmingham, tel. 0121 551 1679. A

small green company supplying fruit and vegetables. They use recyclable bags.

Limited Resources, Manchester, tel. 0161 226 4777. Fruit and vegetables, wholefoods, bread, wine and beer, Traidcraft tea and coffee. They offer a recycling service and delivery by bicycle.

Progress and Nature, Shropshire, Lancashire, Greater Manchester, Merseyside, Wirral and North Wales (tel. 0151 523 6221). Fruit and vegetables, bread, wholefoods and organic eggs.

Beanies, Sheffield, tel. 0114 268 1662. A co-operative, supplying fruit and vegetables in various box sizes. They specialize in organic baby foods. Wholefoods and breads.

Growing with Nature, Preston, Blackburn, Chorley, Lancaster (tel. 01253 790046). Three box sizes. Fruit and vegetables.

The Fresh Food Company, London, tel. 0181 969 0351. Fruit and vegetable box, meat boxes and Cornish fish boxes.

As well as eating organic food, lower your intake of processed foods, including loaves, sugars and drinks, and manipulated fats like margarine.

Stop smoking cigarettes, which contain two gases which make up the greenhouse effect. Cigarettes seriously damage your unborn child's chances of a good quality of life and a healthy childhood as well as damaging your own lungs.

Eat detoxifying foods such as garlic, onions, seaweed and fibres, and ask your doctor for advice on those rich in vitamin C. Take extra detoxifying vitamins in the form of food-state vitamins like B1 and B12 and D and organically bonded minerals rich in calcium, iron, manganese, magnesium and selenium. Look for multivitamin and mineral supplements like Nature's Own (call 01684 892555 for stockists). They produce unique tablets which, through a patented process, have been bonded to food proteins which makes them easy to assimilate. They are recommended and prescribed by many doctors and they have been thoroughly tested.

Garlic can be grown at home. Certified, disease-free garlic for cultivation is obtainable from Jennifer Birch, Garfield Villa, Belle Vue Road, Stroud, Gloucestershire, tel. 01453 750 371.

This section was contributed by Bernadette Vallely, author and broadcaster on green issues, founder and former director of the Women's Environmental Network and editor of Radical Motherhood *magazine.*

Complementary Medicines and Therapies

Most complementary practitioners work on the assumption that everyone is different. Even if two people appear to display identical symptoms, a diagnosis is made only after an examination of an individual's constitutional weaknesses and all possible causes of their complaint. A practitioner needs to understand the patient's emotional make-up as well as her symptoms, medical history, diet and sleep patterns.

Given the confusion over which drugs you can and cannot take during pregnancy, complementary medicines can provide the perfect antidote to the physical and emotional stresses of pregnancy and birth. This section does not cover all complementary therapies, but those that are commonly recommended.

!!! Warning

Anyone can claim to be an 'alternative therapist'. Some of the treatments can have powerful effects and you could harm yourself or your baby if you are not treated by a properly trained professional.

To be on the safe side:

- Always consult your doctor first. He may well practise complementary medicine as well as the more orthodox kind, or he may have a colleague to whom he can refer you on the NHS.
- If you or your baby have symptoms such as a fever or severe pain, consult your doctor immediately. Complementary remedies can always be used if immediate medical attention is not required.
- Where possible, use a practitioner who comes with a strong personal recommendation from someone you trust. Otherwise, see addresses given at the end of this section.

Acupuncture

Acupuncture involves the painless insertion of needles into the skin at pressure points, releasing endorphins (the body's natural painkillers) into the bloodstream. It can be effective in treating pain, arthritis, allergies and menstrual problems. It is thought to be particularly successful in treating physical symptoms caused by emotional stress.

The Council of Acupuncture say that women can be treated for any complications of pregnancy without harm to the mother or baby, although certain pressure points have to be avoided because of the risk of miscarriage.

A GP may be able to refer you or your child on the NHS. If not, contact the British Acupuncture Association, tel. 0171 834 1012, or the British Acupuncture Council on 0181 964 0222.

Reputable practitioners will have had at least two years' training and should belong to the British Acupuncture Council, who will provide a list of practitioners.

Alexander Technique

Alexander practitioners believe that poor posture leads to physical aches and pains and mental problems such as anxiety and a feeling of failure. The technique involves the correction of posture using extremely gentle manipulation and instruction.

To find out about local practitioners and get advice on qualifications to look for, ring the Society for Teachers of Alexander Technique on 0171 351 0828.

If you cannot find a local practitioner the next best thing is the recently published *The Alexander Technique for Pregnancy and Childbirth* by Brita Forsstrom and Mel Hampson (£10.99, published by Victor Gollancz).

Aromatherapy

Aromatherapy is the use of essential oils from certain plants, which are either inhaled or absorbed through the skin. It is often recommended for morning sickness, stretch marks, constipation, postnatal depression and to assist the healing of the perineum after birth.

However, most aromatherapy products should not be used during the first three months of pregnancy and since many mothers' skin becomes sensitive during pregnancy you should test oils on a small patch of skin the day before a treatment even if you have used them before.

Essential oils in the wrong hands can be lethal. There is no legislation controlling the storage or concentration of oils, and information on the labels can be inadequate – there are often no warnings for people with epilepsy, for example.

A number of midwives have completed an approved course in aromatherapy, undergoing five hundred hours of theory and clinical experience. Hitchinbrook Hospital in Cambridge and John Radcliffe Hospital, Oxford, are two well-known centres of excellence. However, *Modern Midwife* magazine warns that some midwives are using aromatherapy in the belief that attendance at a few workshops is sufficient training. And 'how many midwives are aware that there are four different lavenders which have varying effects?' asks *Nursing Times*.

If you live in Middlesex, Mala Morjaria is a qualified midwife and aromatherapist who will give you treatments in your own home. She covers Brent, Harrow and Hillingdon. Call her on 0181 427 2932.

What to look for

- Seventy per cent of oils on the market are not pure essential oils.
- Purer products are always sold in glass bottles as they can damage skin, wood and plastic.
- If the oils are sold without a 'dropper', it is difficult to work out correct doses.
- Light alters the oil, so it should be stored in a dark bottle with a lid that closes securely.
- Buy oils from reputable sources, e.g., Tisserand (telephone 01273 325666 for stockists), Shirley Price (01455 615436), Micheline Arcier (0171 235 3545), or Neal's Yard (0171 498 1686).

Essential Wellbeing offer four product ranges which are safe for mothers-to-be, new mothers and babies. The Labour Day Pack costs £14.99 and the Mother–Baby pack £11.99. These are available from Bumpsadaisy stores or by mail order from Essential Wellbeing, tel. 01734 791737.

Aromatherapy organizations

Amongst the larger organizations to look out for are the International Society of Practising Aromatherapists (ISPA) or the International Federation of Aromatherapists (IFA). For a list of practitioners in your area contact the British Complementary Medicine Association on 01242 226770, or the Aromatherapy Organizations Council, the UK governing body for aromatherapy, on 01858 434242.

Bach Flower Remedies

A system of herbal treatment devised by the British bacteriologist Edward Bach during the 1920s and 1930s. Bach believed that floral remedies could successfully calm negative emotional states like excessive fear as well as the physiological symptoms of illnesses such as schizophrenia.

The most popular item in the flower remedy range is 'Rescue Remedy', a combination of five herbs to be taken in any emergency situation. Call 0171 495 2404 for mail order and stockists.

Chiropractic

Chiropractic is an independent branch of medicine which specializes in the diagnosis and treatment of mechanical joint disorders. It is a mature and rapidly growing profession with proven effectiveness in the treatment of lower-back pain. You can be referred on the NHS if the area health commission or a fund-holding GP has a contract with a local chiropractor. Chiropractic can help with pain caused by accident or injuries; neck pain, arm pain, headaches and leg pain.

Your first visit involves a full examination of individual bones, joints and muscles. X-rays may be necessary. Treatment consists of unlocking stiffness in the joints with skilled hand movements. The BCA (British Chiropractic Association) recognize the following qualifications: DC, B.App.Sci., and B.Sc. (Chiropractic). Telephone the BCA for more information on 01734 757557.

Cranial Osteopathy

This is a gentle manipulation of the skull which is sometimes suggested as a treatment for colic (see Chapter 19). Practitioners must be fully qualified osteopaths. If you are taking your baby for treatment, make sure that the practitioner is experienced in this area. Contact the General Council and Register of Osteopaths on 01734 576585 for further information.

The Osteopathic Centre for Children, 19a Cavendish Square, London W1, tel. 0171 495 1231, is highly reputable.

Herbalism

Most herbal remedies are gentle but they are not harmless and dosage recommendations should be followed precisely.

For a list of qualified herbalists, contact either the General Council and Register of Consultant Herbalists on 01273 680504, or the National Institute of Medical Herbalists, 56 Longbrook Street, Exeter, Devon, EX4 6AH, tel. 01392 426022. If you send the NIMH a self-addressed envelope with a 29p stamp, they will send you an introductory booklet.

It should be pointed out that the NIMH do not recognize the training or qualifications of the General Council and Register of Consultant Herbalists, as its members may lack medical training in anatomy and physiology.

Herbal tips
- Try calendula (marigold) cream for nappy rash.
- Camomile or fennel tea can help with colic.

Homoeopathy

Homoeopaths believe in the principle of treating like with like. Sick people are given minute doses of a drug that would create the symptoms of their disease in a healthy person. Some GPs practise homoeopathy alongside conventional medicine.

Although there are many books available on how to use homoeopathic remedies at home, you should really see an expert. You have to be able to recognize all your symptoms to prescribe the right treatment.

For further information, contact the Society of Homoeopaths,

2 Artisan Road, Northampton NN1 4HU, tel. 01604 21400.

Homoeopathic remedies are available from large chemists and the following offer next-day delivery: Ainsworths, 36 New Cavendish Street, London W1M 7LH, tel. 0171 935 5330, or Helios, 97 Camden Road, Tunbridge Wells, Kent TN1 2QR, tel. 01892 536393. Both have a twenty-four-hour answerphone service.

Hypnosis

Hypnosis can be used to control pain and can help women through labour. Hypnotherapists can teach self-hypnotic techniques, ways of inducing in-depth relaxation or deep trance states.

Expert Douglas Simmons says that the time to consider hypnosis is well before labour. 'As childbirth is a painful procedure, one can only expect to be in agony, but most of this is due to fear. Hypnosis can correct these preconceived ideas by reframing them through learning breathing techniques and hypnotic patterns, going through a mental rehearsal of the birth and learning how to handle pain.' If you are considering using hypnosis to give up smoking now that you are pregnant, Simmons suggests: 'Hypnosis is good when used in conjunction with other techniques. You have to discover if smoking is a crutch, the reasons why somebody smokes. Otherwise you will take away this crutch and the subject will simply find another.'

Many hypnotherapists are practising doctors who use the technique in combination with orthodox forms of treatment. The danger of going to a lay hypnotherapist is that he may be incorrect in his initial diagnosis of your problems and may then treat you incorrectly.

A list of qualified hypnotherapists is available from the UK College for Complementary Healthcare Studies, St Charles Hospital, Exmoor Street, London W10 6DZ, tel. 0181 964 1206. Alternatively, leave a message on the answering machine at the

British Hypnotherapy Association, 1 Wythburn Place, London W1H 5WL, tel. 0171 723 4443.

Hypnosis in childbirth

Hypnosis involves a very personal relationship between the therapist and his patient, which means that your own therapist, and not just any doctor, has to be available at a moment's notice and for long periods once labour begins. This is time-consuming and difficult to arrange unless the therapist also happens to be your obstetrician or midwife.

Massage

Almost anyone can give a massage and nearly every pregnancy book recommends that a pregnant woman's partner should become a masseur during pregnancy and labour. If you fancy a back massage but find it too uncomfortable to lie on your front, sit astride a chair, supporting the front of your body with cushions. Leg and foot massage are also wonderfully relaxing.

Reflexology

It has long been recognized that the internal organs are represented on the surface of the body by areas of skin that share the same nerve supplies as these organs. A condition in the diaphragm will produce pain in the shoulder simply because they share the same nerve supply. Certain reflex points on the foot are believed to influence other organs of the body and stroking or pressing them is said to stimulate these areas or to relieve the tension in them.

You are unlikely to get reflexology on the NHS. For the address of a reflexologist in your area who is on the British register, write enclosing a large SAE to the Institute of Complementary Medicine, PO Box 194, London SE16 1QZ, tel. 0171 237 5165.

Your Baby and the Environment

Generally parents treat newborn babies with the utmost respect and avoid all forms of chemical and toxic pollution that can be harmful to them. However, there are many products which, although safe in themselves, are manufactured in a way which causes pollution.

Green Nappies

Disposable nappies are a major source of enrivonmental pollution. Reusable nappies are far cheaper, take up fewer resources in their manufacture and involve less waste and pollution. They don't rely on cutting down forests or the dubious chemicals used to produce the paper pulp which makes up the largest ingredient in a conventional disposable nappy. The manufacture of so-called 'super-absorbent nappies' involves a polyacrylite chemical which has been tested on animals and the plastic which surrounds the nappy will probably last for several hundred, if not thousands of years in a landfill site. Disposable nappies make up around 4 per cent of UK household waste and we throw away eight tons of them each hour, every day.

Nappy-washing services are available now if you can't face the idea of washing your own nappies – there are about seventy of them operating in the UK at present. Call the National Association of Nappy Services (NANS), St George House, Hill Street, Birmingham B5 4AN, tel. 0121 693 4949, for an idea of what is offered in your area.

For a list of stockists of reusable nappies, see Chapter 10.

Green Toiletries

Cleaning powders, soaps and wipes might look completely safe, soft and gentle, but some of them contain hidden chemicals, including perfumes and bleaches. These are mostly unnecessary and may cause allergic reactions. Many have been tested on animals and some include animal-based products like lanolin from sheep, which can be contaminated by organochlorine chemicals used in sheep-dip. Some companies specifically avoid lanolin and instead use hypoallergenic ingredients, clean enough to satisfy medical standards. Avoid using cleaners and chemicals in your baby's bath. Often you need no more than a sponge or face flannel to clean a child, and you do not need to use shampoo every time you wash his hair.

If your nipples are sore or dry, use olive oil instead of creams that contain lanolin.

The following products are not tested on animals:

Body Shop Mama Toto, available from Body Shop International plc, Watersmead, Little Hampton, West Sussex BN17 6LS, tel. 01903 731500, or from branches nationwide. A range of baby toiletries including corn-based baby powder and baby oil. All products contain natural ingredients and are suitable for vegans.

The Weleda Calendula Baby Care range, from Weleda UK (Ltd), Heanor Road, Ilkeston, Derbyshire DE7 8DR, tel. 01159 448200, is based on organic plant ingredients. Weleda also offer herbal toothpastes, including plant-gel paste for children. Products are available by mail order or from some health-food stores and chemists.

Elysia Lindos Camomile Baby toiletries, from Elysia Natural Skin Care, Haselor, College Road, Bromsgrove, West Midlands DY9 9PX, tel. 01527 832863, include soap, shampoo and nappy cream made from organic-plant ingredients. They are manufactured with the minimum environmental impact. Contact the above number for a list of retail outlets or to place an order.

Bodywise Natracare Vegan toiletries are vegan baby care products available from health stores and selected pharmacies.

Kingfisher Natural Toothpaste, 21 White Lodge Estate, Hall Road, Norwich NR4 6DG, tel. 01603 630484. The range includes children's strawberry-flavoured toothpaste which is vegan and free from artificial substances and animal testing. It is available in supermarkets and health-food shops.

Green Clothes

Supplying clothes for children is a continuous process, so don't waste the opportunity to save on resources and money by thinking about ways of recycling clothes. Friends and relatives with children are the obvious first source of second-hand clothes for your baby: children grow so quickly that often these can be virtually unworn. The cheapest places to buy by far are traditional jumble sales, but there are also many shops around the country that swap clothes or act as an agency by selling them for you for a fee of 50 per cent of the ticket price.

Baby on a Budget by Noelle Walsh (Pan, £3.99), lists second-hand baby-clothes shops nationwide.

If you want to buy new items look out for natural fibres which absorb sweat effectively, are made from renewable resources and are more hard-wearing. Schmidt Natural Clothing, 155 Tuffley Lane, Gloucester GL4 0NZ, tel. 01452 416016, sell nappy trial packs, knitted cotton wraparounds, vests, blankets and towels made of wool or cotton.

For clothes which are a little bit different, **Carlsen**, 8 Heath Drive, Sulton, Surrey SM2 5RP, tel. 0181 642 9266, produce distinctive knitwear in natural fibres, and **Polly Flinders**, Lower House, Sarn, Newton, Powys SY16 4EL, offer hand-painted, machine-washable styles at affordable prices.

US Kids, Chaldon, Ellesmere Road, Weybridge, Surrey KT13 0HS, tel. 01932 840412, supply clothing for 0–4-year-olds. **Cotton Moon Ltd** (NG5), Freepost (SE8265), PO Box 280, London SE3 8BR, tel: 0181 319 8315, have generously cut American-style clothing for children from six months to six years. They are 100 per cent cotton, 100 per cent washable and 100 per cent comfortable.

Green Equipment

Hundreds of pounds are often spent on completely unnecessary gadgets and space-consuming furniture. Ask other parents what they found useful and why, and what they wouldn't buy again and why. Think ecology when you purchase equipment, and buy second-hand whenever you can. Go to jumble sales and look in newspaper small ads for cots, buggies and prams. Consider using slings and wraps to carry your baby, especially in the first crucial months while you are bonding. When buying a cot mattress, remember that PVC and foam fillings are made by a process which includes organochlorines.

The following sell environmentally friendly equipment:

Baby futons, three layers of cotton fibre in a 100 per cent cotton cover, are available from the **Healthy House**, Cold Harbour, Ruscombe, Stroud GL6 6DA, tel. 01453 752216.

Nippers UK Franchising Ltd, Mansers, Nizels Lane, Hildenborough, Kent TN11 8NX, offer new and second-hand baby equipment and toys.

Kiddycare, Easter Lawrenceton, Forres, Scotland IV36 0RL, tel. 01309 674646, sell baby sleeping-bags, a kind of cross between a sleeping-bag and a babygro, which keep babies warm and comfortable.

The Huggababy, an easy-to-use sling suitable for babies from birth up to eighteen months, is available from **Huggababy**, The Baby Carrier, Dept NG4, 40b Haringey Park, London N8 9JD, tel. 0181 292 6030. Other varieties are sold by the **Better Baby Sling Company**, 60 Sumatra Road, London NW6 1PR, tel. 0171 433 3727.

Green Toys

Avoid plastic toys – they are more polluting to manufacture than other kinds and they can sometimes contain solvents. As your child grows, the likelihood of her developing an affection for battery-operated toys will increase. Far more energy is used in the production of batteries than you ever get from the battery itself, and they contain huge amounts of toxic chemicals. Opt for wind-up toys instead, or those which don't need propelling at all – after all, children will play with almost anything, including pots and pans, food and scraps.

Many toys are made with the environment in mind, including those whose manufacturers use raw materials from sustainable sources. Look for the Good Wood Seal of Approval from Friends of the Earth or the World Wildlife Fund-approved logo (WWF).

Outlets for products and services

The Natural Collection Catalogue, mail order, run by Friends of the Earth, tel. 01672 542266.

The **Early Learning Centre**, South Marston Park, Swindon SN3 4TJ, tel. 01793 444844, or branches nationwide.

Traidcraft, Kingsway, Team Valley Trading Estate, Gateshead, Tyne and Wear NE11 0NE, tel. 0191 491 0591.

Playring, 53 Westbere Road, London NW6, tel. 0171 794 9497. Really nice wooden toys for babies and toddlers. They sell the Squish from Canada, a textural rattly toy guaranteed to provide hours of amusement (also available by mail order from **Babybasics** on 01703 234949, price £12.50).

Garden Designs with your Child in Mind, Heather Marsh, tel. 0114 258 6838. Have your garden designed as a safe, stimulating environment where your child can learn and play.

Helpful organizations

The **Women's Environmental Network** is a non-profit-making organization committed to empowering women who care about the planet. Literature is available on a wide range of subjects including nappies, tobacco, parenting, green consumerism. They run a free information hotline service called **WENDi** (tel. 0171 704 6800) and they can be reached at

22 Highbury Grove, London N5 2EA, tel. 0171 354 8823.

The **Natural Nurturing Network** aims to explore and encourage ways of lovingly and respectfully nurturing our children, ourselves and each other, true to our nature as a carrying species and an innately social animal. Membership costs £7 for one year, which includes a quarterly newsletter and address list of members. Also available from the network is a directory of organizations with similar aims and views, a booklet containing a list of books and other publications recommended by members as helpful, inspirational or supportive, a compilation of book reviews and a number of articles on relevant subjects. For further information contact Elspeth Campbell, PO Box 3162, Sherington, Bucks MK16 9XS.

Further reading

Natural Childhood: A Practical Guide to the First Seven Years by John B. Thomson, Gaia Books, £14.99.

Green Babies by Dr Penny Stanway, Random Century, £9.99.

Home Ecology by Karen Christensen, Arlington Books, £6.95.

Green Parenting by Juliet Solomon, Optima, £6.99.

The Vegetarian Society Guide to Nutrition During Pregnancy and Beyond, available from the Vegetarian Society, Parkdale, Dunham Road, Altrincham, Cheshire WA14 4QG.

The Ecological Impact of Bottle Feeding by Andrew Radford. A briefing available from Baby Milk Action, tel. 01223 464420.

The Politics of Breastfeeding by Gabrielle Palmer, Pandora, £6.95.

Planning for a Healthy Baby by Belinda Barnes and Suzanne Gail Bradley, Ebury Press, £6.95.

Mothers Know Best, a new monthly newsletter from the editors of *What Doctors Don't Tell You*. Includes letters, articles on a variety of topics from home schooling to advertising. The contributing editor is Deborah Jackson. A year's subscription is £24.95. For further information, contact Mothers Know Best, 4 Wallace Road, London N1 2PG, tel. 0171 354 4592.

Radical Motherhood magazine offers information on a wide range of ecologically conscious and political subjects for parents, including vaccination, hemp and marijuana, depression and herbal help and tantric sex after childbirth. Send £2.50 for a sample issue to Radical Motherhood, 60 Osbaldeston Road, London N16 7DR.

This section was contributed by Bernadette Vallely, author and broadcaster on green issues, founder and former director of the Women's Environmental Network and editor of Radical Motherhood *magazine.*

PART THREE
GIVING BIRTH

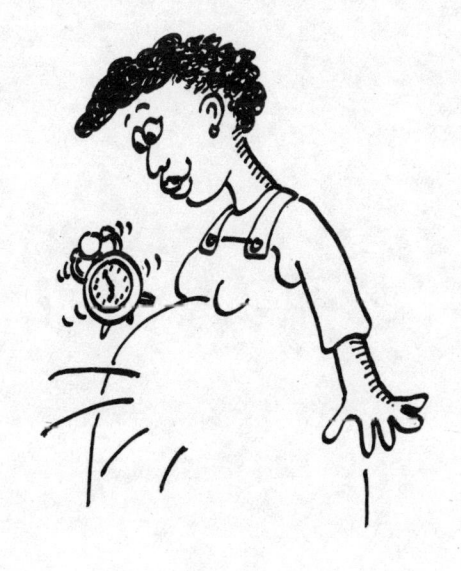

7 The Big Day

Birth Plans

'Just tear the bloody thing up and keep me free of pain!'
Quoted by a midwife recalling a recent birth

The most important aspect of labour is that your baby is delivered safely and in good health. You must trust your carers to help you achieve this. Your own birth 'experience' must come second to the needs of your baby. However, you may wish to establish at an early stage the way you would ideally like your labour to be managed.

Cathy McCormick, midwifery liaison manager at the Royal College of Midwives, must be one of Britain's experts when it comes to birth plans. Her advice is this:

- A birth plan must be developed by the parents along with the professionals who will be with them during labour.
- Write down what you *think* you would like to happen and then talk it through with the midwife or doctor.
- You need to know the consequences of any specific request you might make.
- You must remember that labour is a dynamic occurrence and that you cannot plan it in tablets of stone.
- You must be prepared for dramatic alterations to your plan – it *will* change and it *will* have to be adapted.

Writing Your Birth Plan

Keep it brief and flexible – there may not be time to read through pages of instructions. Headings you might consider are:

- **Birth companions.** Who will be accompanying you? This is particularly important if it is someone other than the baby's father.
- **People in the room.** Do you mind if students are present? If not, would you rather that there was a limited number?
- **Birth pools.** Do you want to use one if it is available?
- **Positions for labour and delivery.** You may feel you would like to squat or kneel on all fours, but you will only know this once you are in the throes of labour. You might write something like: 'I would like to be encouraged to try different positions to assist delivery, e.g., squatting.'
- **Pain relief.** Keep your options open. If you are keen to avoid drugs, write something along the lines of: 'I would like to manage without drugs, but if I change my mind, please help me to choose a suitable form of pain relief.'
- **Cuts and tears.** You will need to discuss this question in advance. Some hospitals are more persistent about episiotomies than others. The Avon Episiotomy Support Group is a voluntary organization hoping to form a support network for mothers. For information, write to them at PO Box 130, Weston-Super-Mare, Avon BS23 4YJ.
- **Aspects of delivery you feel very strongly about.** If there are things you really want – for example, to be consulted about intervention, for your partner to cut the cord, or the baby to be cleaned and wrapped before he or she is given to you – say so. Similarly, if there are things that would really upset you, make this clear.
- **Consider special circumstances.** If, for example, you have to have a Caesarean, think about the implications. State: 'I would like my partner to stay with me if I need a Caesarean', or 'I will still be keen to breastfeed on demand.'

Choices for Pain Relief

It is rare for women to experience no pain in labour, but fortunately there are so many methods of pain relief that one is bound to work for you. Because most labours start gradually, you should have time to acclimatize yourself to how it feels and decide as you go along what level of relief you need, whether it is simply the relaxation of a massage or the total freedom from pain offered by an epidural.

You may think you want a 'natural' birth, but if in the event you do not have one, it is not a sign of failure; it is a question of mature adults making the right decisions to safeguard the health of both mother and baby.

Walking around and finding different positions to sit or lie in can help alleviate pain. You can also use some of the following.

Breathing Techniques

You have to find someone to teach you these in advance. Some antenatal classes do this as part of their programme.

PLUS POINTS
* The more relaxed you are, the less likely you are to feel pain.
* Good breathing technique can relax the muscles needed to push out the baby, making intervention less likely.
* The labour feels under your control.
* As drugs are not involved, there are no side-effects. However, consider combining breathing techniques with other methods of pain relief.

MINUS POINT
* In the heat of the moment you may forget everything you have learned. Practising with your birth companion prior to labour is a great help.

Water

If your hospital does not have facilities for water births, you can hire a birthing pool for use at home or in hospital. You will need written consent from the director of midwifery services to bring a portable pool into the hospital.

If you have set your heart on a water birth but cannot find one locally and have some spare cash, you might consider paying an independent midwife to assist your labour. Send an A5 SAE to the Independent Midwives Association, Nightingale Cottage, Shamblehurst Lane, Botley SO32 2BY. They can send you a list of experienced water-birth midwives. Expect to pay around £1,000. This will obviously vary depending on where you live and whether the midwife looks after you throughout your antenatal and postnatal period. Some midwives have their own portable birthing pools; others will ask you to hire one.

PLUS POINTS
* Buoyancy can relieve back problems.
* Because it relaxes you, it can speed up a labour which has slowed down.

MINUS POINTS
* Most midwives will insist on a period of monitoring before you are allowed into the pool, so you will need to decide well in advance that you want to try water.
* If your baby needs constant monitoring, you may not be able to get into the birthing pool.
* It cannot be combined with all pain-relief options, e.g. certain drugs, and TENS (see page 142).
* Some doctors believe that if you give birth in the water your baby may inhale contaminated water.
* Your midwife may find it difficult to assist in the event of a sudden complication like bleeding before the baby is born.

Which type of pool?

You need to decide if you want an inflatable pool or one with hard sides. Hard-sided pools allow you to brace yourself against the walls to push. Remember that when they are full, pools are heavy. Check the weight before taking delivery – your floor may not be able to cope.

All the firms seem to offer something slightly different. Birthworks, for example, supply cleansing tablets so that you do not have to change the water. This may be of interest if you intend to spend a few days using the pool before labour. Some pools come with heaters, but your midwife may think that an unnecessary expense. Ask her advice before committing yourself.

Pool-hire companies

Aqua Pools, Active Birth Centre, 25 Bickerton Road, London N19 5JT, tel. 0171 561 9006. Hire from £21 per week; delivery from £25 (flat fee for small pool), £50 for large pool, anywhere in the UK.

Birthworks, Unit 4E, Brent Mill Trading Estate, Lond Meadow, South Brent, Devon TQ10 9YT, tel. 01364 72802. Hire from £15 per week; delivery £50 anywhere in the UK.

Blue Lagoon, Beacon House, Woodley Park, Skelmersdale, Lancashire WN8 6UR, tel. 01695 556642. Minimum of three weeks' hire (£162) for those within a fifty-mile radius of Bolton or Skelmersdale. This includes delivery and set-up in your home or the hospital and all necessary kit. They will deliver elsewhere, but charges may differ. Ring for details.

Splashdown Water Birth Services, 17 Wellington Terrace, Harrow-on-the-Hill, Middlesex HA1 3EP, tel. 0181 422 9308. Hire is £115, inclusive of all equipment, plus £20 delivery charge anywhere in the UK.

You can also ring your local NCT branch and ask if there is anyone in the area who supplies pools. Water births are growing hugely in popularity and there may well be a new pool-hire company on your doorstep.

Massage

Particularly helpful during the first stage of labour.

> **PLUS POINTS**
> * No side-effects.
> * Pressure helps deal with pain and aids relaxation.
>
> **MINUS POINT**
> * You need someone there to do it for you, and they may find it exhausting.

Transcutaneous Electrical Nerve Stimulation (TENS)

TENS is a small, portable battery pack that links to electrodes placed on your back. It generates electrical impulses which interfere with your body's pain signals and stimulate the natural painkillers in your body, the endorphins. You can control the electrical impulses according to the strength of the contractions.

At your later health check-ups, it is essential for your midwife or doctor to mark in *pen* on your back where the electrodes should be positioned. If they are put in the wrong place, TENS may not work.

> **PLUS POINTS**
> * You are controlling your own level of pain relief.
> * You can start using TENS at home before going into hospital for delivery.
> * It can be combined with some other pain relief methods, e.g., gas and air.
>
> **MINUS POINTS**
> * You may dislike the tingly feeling.
> * Positioned wrongly, it may not work at all.

Complementary Therapies *(see Chapter 6)*

PLUS POINT
* If you can use your own expertise or that of your midwife, pain relief is inexpensive and non-invasive.

MINUS POINTS
* Therapies should only be undertaken with expert advice.
* Having an additional practitioner at the birth would be expensive and you would need written permission from the director of midwifery services to bring someone into the hospital.
* They can take too long to work.
* They may not give enough relief.

Entonox (Gas and Air)

This is a mixture of oxygen and nitrous oxide which you inhale through a mask.

PLUS POINTS
* You can still move around.
* Entonox is not thought to cause any side-effects.
* You are in control of the amount you take.

MINUS POINTS
* It may make you feel nauseous or light-headed.
* It does not offer total pain relief.

Pethidine

This is a strong pain-relieving drug given by injection.

PLUS POINT
* Can make you feel detached and relaxed.

MINUS POINTS
* Pethidine may make you feel nauseous.
* It may affect the baby's breathing or ability to feed, though the baby will be given an antidote injection if this happens.

Meptid (Metazinol)

This drug is similar to Pethidine, but you control the amount you take. It is not thought to affect the baby to the same extent as Pethidine. You will probably not be offered this, but most hospitals have it if you ask.

Epidural

A local anaesthetic which partially or completely numbs the body below the waist. Have it as early as possible as it takes a while to set up – especially if the ward is busy. Mobile epidurals are available in some hospitals, enabling you to walk around if you want to.

PLUS POINTS
* The most effective method of total pain relief.
* It can be adjusted, so you can indicate to the anaesthetist how much you want to feel.
* The reduction in pain leaves you free to relax and enjoy labour – in some hospitals they will wheel in a television.
* Can help high blood pressure.
* If you suddenly need a Caesarean, your epidural is simply topped up and you remain wide awake for the birth.

MINUS POINTS
* You will be put on a drip at the same time to stop a fall in blood pressure.
* You may be one of the small group of women for whom an epidural does not work.
* There is an increased likelihood of intervention because you cannot feel yourself pushing. You can always ask for the epidural to be allowed to wear off at the end of the first stage so that you regain your ability to feel.
* Occasionally there are side-effects, such as a severe headache.
* The loss of feeling in your legs is a strange sensation.

Spinal Block

An effective local anaesthetic that may be used for an assisted delivery by forceps or ventouse.

General Anaesthetic

This makes you totally unconscious and is normally only used if an emergency Caesarean section is required.

What to Pack for Hospital

For You

You may find it helpful to put your 'labour gear' at the top of the bag or in a separate one from the items you need later on.

Labour

Birth plan
Long baggy T-shirt or nightshirt — Useful for wandering around in during the first stage of labour. Wear a hospital gown (if anything) for the actual delivery. Why mess up your own clothes?

Cardigan or dressing gown
Slippers or non-slip socks — Your feet can get very cold during labour so soft slippers or warm socks may come in useful.

Walkman and tapes
Snack/drink in carton with a straw — Check with midwife that this is allowed.
Small Evian spray or thermos of cold water and flannel — Your birth partner can use these to cool your face during the last stages of labour.

After labour

Towel and a toilet bag	Some wonderful-smelling soap or spray is an antidote to the clinical environment.
Disinfectant and a sponge	If you are desperate for a bath and dislike showers, you will need these to give the bath a good once-over before you get in it.
Make-up	If you normally wear make-up, you will regret not having it for the postnatal photo sessions.
At least two front-opening nighties	For breastfeeding. Bring in as much washable nightwear as you can, as you will want to change frequently.
Three to six pairs of NCT stretch pants or Mothercare disposable knickers	These hold maternity pads/ice packs in place. At £4 for three they are neither cheap nor elegant, but they are very comfortable and can be hand-washed in moments and dried on a radiator. They will last for more than one delivery and can be worn above or below a section scar. Telephone 0141 6335552 to order. Disposable knickers will save extra washing when you get home.
Nursing bras and breast pads	You may want some cabbage leaves and nipple cream too (see pages 239–40).
Maternity/heavy-flow sanitary pads	Do not buy the 'winged' variety if you are using disposable knickers – they will tear the pants.
Earplugs and eyeshades (free from some airlines)	The noise and light in the ward can keep you awake when you are desperate to sleep.
Change for phone or phonecard	
Stamps, writing paper, pen, scissors	You will be surprised what you need.
Clothes to come home in	Anything that fitted you when you were six months' pregnant.

For Your Partner

Camera and film

Change of shirt and toilet bag — He may be there for many hours and a freshen-up can work wonders.

Book or newspaper — It is unlikely that he will have a moment but you never know.

Food — Two large snacks will probably get eaten.

Phonecard or change for payphone

Names and numbers of people to call

For the Baby

Four stretch suits
Cardigan
First-sized nappies
Cotton wool or newborn wipes
Towel
Shawl or cellular cotton blanket
Outerwear to go home in
Baby carrier for the car

Premature Babies

You are bound to be in a state of shock if your baby appears before it is expected. Dramatic improvements in medical care mean that the majority of early babies will be fine: Britain's most premature baby to survive was born 122 days early and weighed 1lb 3oz. Of all babies born, one in ten need special care, and one in fifty needs intensive care.

Nearly all babies born between thirty-two and thirty-four weeks are taken into the special-care baby unit (SCBU). It can be deeply distressing to see your baby lying in an incubator connected to so many tubes. If you know that there is a risk of your baby arriving early:

- Prepare yourselves by visiting the SCBU ahead of time.
- When you are there, find out what all the equipment is for. If you are familiar with it, it will not be so upsetting when you see your own baby in an incubator.

The SCBU will have monitoring equipment for his heart rate, breathing and blood pressure. You should be prepared to see a tube up his nose or in his mouth attached to a ventilator to assist his breathing. Chest X-rays will be taken and oxygen levels in the blood will also be measured. If your baby has jaundice, which is extremely common, he will be given light treatment, phototherapy, for which he will wear eye pads to protect his eyes from the light.

The golden rule

If anything particularly worries you, ask for explanations until you get answers that satisfy you.

Paid Maternity Leave

Legally, a premature baby is regarded no differently to a full-term baby. Although you have no automatic rights to extend your leave, you could ask either for unpaid leave or to take some of your holiday entitlement when your maternity leave is up.

Feeding Your Baby

Most hospitals will encourage you to express breast milk. The SCBU will have facilities for storing it until your baby needs it. If you only produce tiny amounts, do not be downhearted: your baby will probably not require large quantities. If you cannot produce anything worthwhile, there are specially designed premature baby milks. Try to be involved with feeding your baby as soon as it is possible – even very small babies are thought to respond differently when their mother touches them.

Clothes and Nappies

Do not use dolls' clothes because:
- They do not wash well.
- They could be restrictive owing to their small collars and armholes.
- Badly finished buttons and sharp zips make them unsafe for real babies.

Mothercare, Adams, Woolworth and Children's World all sell smaller baby clothes but it is worth ringing in advance to see what your local branch has in stock as the range may be limited. Sewing patterns for dungarees and dresses are available from the Neonatal Unit, City Hospital, Hucknall Road, Nottingham NG5 1PB. Knitting patterns are available from BLISS at the address below. Please send a large SAE.

Boots have 'pre-mini' nappies up to 6lb (3kg), and Pampers do micro-nappies for 2 to 8lb babies.

You can buy mail-order clothes for premature babies from the following:

Tiddlywinks, tel. 01943 878843. A full range of clothes for babies from 2lb (1kg).

Tiny Trends, tel. 01202 523060. Sizes start at 2½lb (1.5kg).

Babycare Dollycare, tel. 0116 2773013. A full range from 3lb (2kg).

Pretty Small, tel. 0191 2641813.

Helpful organizations

BLISS (Baby Life Support Systems), 17–21 Emerald Street, London WC1N 3QL, tel. 0171 831 9393 or Mercury Freecall 0500 151617. Founded in 1979, BLISS is Britain's leading charity for newborn babies. Its aim is to give every baby an equal chance in its start in life. Much of the equipment in the UK's special-care baby units is funded by BLISS with donations from companies and individuals. The organization also sponsors specialist nurse training and offers support to parents whose babies need special care at birth.

The BLISS Guide to Neonatal Equipment is a booklet with photographs and simple explanations of the equipment used in SCBUs. Send an A4 SAE to BLISS for a free copy. Another booklet, *Going Home – Taking Your Special-Care Baby Home*, answers virtually every question you will have on the subject.

The **NCT** (0181 992 8637) will give you a list of support groups in your area.

In addition, your local SCBU may have its own support group.

Parents of Prems (POPs) give support to parents whose babies need any form of neonatal care. Tel. 0121 326 9085.

Parent Information Network and Support (POPPINS) offers support to families whose children have learning difficulties or physical impairment following a period of neonatal care. Tel. 0121 778 3482. They provide a range of publications and products that may interest all parents of premature babies.

Remember that you will not be deserted by the medical profession. Community nurses will come round to help and advise.

Toiletries for Postnatal Mothers

Coping with Sore Stitches

The Valley cushion, which allows you to sit down without putting pressure on your stitches, can be hired from your local branch of the NCT. Otherwise, a child's rubber ring in a pillowcase or a piece of foam with a hole cut out of the centre can be slid into a pillowcase to provide a cheap and effective alternative.

Arnica cream (£3.15), a soothing ointment which aids healing and relieves bruising, is good for tears and stitches immediately after the birth.

Sore Muscles

A hot or cold compress is useful for relieving soreness and stiff muscles. This can be bought as part of the Boots first-aid kit or as a separate item (price £4.99). Put it into the microwave or the freezer, depending on whether you want heating up or cooling down. The BooBoo wrap, a reusable cold compress that you store in the fridge, is aimed at accident-prone toddlers, hence the name. It is available from Bright Start mail order (0171 483 3929) at £6.95.

Nipple Creams

Some people recommend that you start rubbing in cream during the last weeks of pregnancy to prepare the nipples for feeding.

At £4.16, Rotasept spray is considered a star buy by many breastfeeding mothers to heal cracked nipples. However, remember to wash it off before feeding.

Maternity Pads

You will probably experience heavy vaginal bleeding immediately following the birth. This will gradually lighten and should stop altogether around six weeks afterwards. Tampons should not be used because of the risk of infection. You can buy special maternity pads from Boots, but they are not necessary.

★★★ Star buys ★★★
Superdrug Options Night-Time press-on towels, £1.10 for ten. These are good value and very absorbent.

8 Registration and Celebration

Registering Your Baby's Birth

You have a legal obligation to register your baby's birth within forty-two days of the delivery. If you are lucky, the registrar will come to the hospital – ask your midwife if this still happens. Otherwise you will have to go to the local register office.

If your baby is born in England and Wales you can register the birth in any register office in England or Wales. The birth certificates and the baby's medical card for registering with your GP will be sent on by post. At the registration you will be given a short certificate, which covers most ordinary needs. A full birth certificate and further short ones can be bought on the spot or at a later date.

If you were married to the father at the time of birth, he can register it on his own. If you were unmarried, the father's details will *not* be entered unless:

- Both mother and father attend together to register the birth.
- The father does not attend but fills in a statutory declaration acknowledging paternity of the child. Copies of the declaration form are available at all register offices. The mother will also have to make a declaration at the time of registration.
- The father and mother have a parental responsibility agree-

ment or court order which can be given to the registrar. (Contact your Citizens' Advice Bureau or a solicitor for details.) In this case only one parent will need to be present.

If the mother cannot attend, she will need to fill in a statutory declaration form, which the father takes along to the registration, where he makes the declaration.

It is important that the information recorded is correct. If you make a mistake, or want to change your child's name, write within twelve months to: Corrections Section, General Register Office, Smedley Hydro, Trafalgar Road, Birkdale, Southport PR8 2HH, or telephone 0151 471 4200 (England and Wales only). In Scotland, contact: Corrections Section, General Register Office for Scotland, New Register House, 3 West Register Street, Edinburgh EH1 3YT, tel. 0131 334 0380.

The information required

Mother: Full name and name before marriage (if applicable); date of marriage (if applicable); place and date of birth; address; occupation; number of previous children.
Father: Full name; place and date of birth; occupation.
Baby: Place and date of birth. In the case of multiple births, the time of each baby's birth; sex of baby; baby's full name.

If you lose the birth certificate, you can get a duplicate from the office where the birth was registered. A copy will cost £5.50 in England and Wales and £10 in Scotland. A duplicate can also be sent from the main register offices listed above but this is more expensive – £15 in England and Wales and £12 in Scotland. The Public Search Room at St Catherine's House, 10 Kingsway, London WC2B 6JP holds details of all births since 1837.

Choosing Your Baby's Name

You will probably find a good book on baby names in your local library, but just in case it was published a few years ago, and you want a name that is different without being outrageous, here is an update on some of the more fashionable names around.

The Times points out that although *The Guinness Book of Names* calculates that 1995's most popular names were Daniel and Rebecca, its author believes 'names that appear top in *The Times* often appear high up on the national lists a few years later because of aspirational naming'. Charlotte is an example.

British names are most commonly drawn from the following sources: The Bible, e.g. Sarah, David; saints, e.g. Anthony, Christopher, Catherine; British tradition, e.g. William, Emma; Celtic tradition, Kevin, Bronwen; films and books, e.g. Olivia, Scarlett, Wayne, Gary; flowers and gems, e.g. Daisy, Jade.

Always consider whether you will be giving your child a set of initials that spell something unfortunate. The name should also go well with the baby's surname. It may not matter to you, but it could be a constant irritant to your child if you give her a name that other people find hard to pronounce or spell. Similarly, a babyish name may become a source of embarrassment later.

Parents are less hidebound when naming daughters. Charlotte's victory was a surprise since she was lagging well behind last year before putting on a spurt.

Top names

1	Thomas		1	Charlotte
2	James		2	Sophie
3	Alexander		3	Emily
4	William		4	Olivia
5	Oliver		5	Alice
6	George		6	Eleanor
7	Charles		7	Elizabeth
8	Henry		8	Lucy
9	Edward		9	Hannah
10	Jack		10	Isabella

This compilation by Lucy Berrington and Alan Hamilton is reproduced courtesy of The Times.

Ceremonies to Mark the Birth

Many parents wish to gather together family and friends to express their joy and commitment to their new baby. You may want to organize a religious ceremony or non-religious ceremony and/or a party.

Traditional Baby Blessing Outfits

If you are looking for an heirloom, **NCT** mail order has a special christening gown design service (prices from £50). Call 0141 633 5552 for details. Otherwise they offer a choice of two nightgowns at £8.50. You can buy nightgowns from **Mothercare** for as little as £4.95.

Clair de Lune produce special christening gowns which can be ordered through a nursery retailer. Ask your local nursery retailer to get hold of the catalogue (tel. 0161 283 4477) as the company does not deal directly with the public. You can hire christening gowns to fit babies up to eighteen months old from Linda Forsey of **Little Treasures**. Telephone 0113 2892720 for details. Prices range from £20 to £60 for the full get-up, including gown and coat in dupion silk. **Heirlooms** mail order (01634 402079) has christening wear starting at £18.

Mail order Mini Boden (tel. 0181 964 2662) also has suitable nighties for £24 and a boy's navy christening suit for £30.

Religious Ceremonies

Contact your minister as soon as you have decided on a religious ceremony. Most congregations will be offered one or a choice of the following:
- A baby blessing as part of the weekly service. If this is the only option, fix a date as soon as possible to ensure that you can arrange a day that suits the majority of your guests.
- A private service for your family and friends.

- A blessing service for a number of families and their new babies.

Fees are not usually charged, but a donation to your place of worship or a related charity may be expected. You might have to pay for a blessing certificate if you want one: check this when you book the ceremony.

Celebration Books (tel. 01428 727645) produce personalized Church of England and Catholic versions of the Bible in bonded white leather with gold or silver print and edging. Prices start at £12.99.

Non-Religious Ceremonies

A secular ceremony offers you a way of celebrating the birth in a way that suits you, and there is no pressure on the parents to be married. Religion need not be mentioned but music or readings from any faith can be included – the choice is yours. Even if you are only vaguely interested in this option, contact Rosie Styles at the Baby-Naming Society, 66 High Street, Pershore, WR10 1DU, tel./fax 01386 555599. She can provide sample ceremonies and readings that will move the iciest of hearts and can write a tailor-made ceremony to suit your requirements. If you are lucky, she may still have a few copies left of her excellent book *How to make a Family Covenant – Child Welcoming Ceremonies*, a DIY guide priced at £4.95. Her new volume will probably be even better, but may not be out for a while.

Parties

Your budget will probably determine the scale of the celebration so you will need to tot up the costs of the following and then decide what you really need.
- Venue.
- Invitations/programmes/thank-you cards plus postage.
- Baby outfit.

- New outfits for other members of the family.
- Flowers.
- Photography/video.
- Catering: food, drink, cake.

Stationery

If you have access to a word-processor or are remotely artistic, there is nothing to stop you generating your own designs for photocopying on to card or paper. If you have to pay for each photocopy in a local shop, you can halve the cost by ensuring that at least two of the cards fit on to one A4 sheet. All machines can photocopy on both sides of one piece of paper. You could decorate each invitation with a photo of the baby, ribbons or using a metallic pen to make them more festive.

If you want to buy stationery, there is a great deal to choose from. Start by browsing in W. H. Smith. If your local stationer stocks the Waverley range, you will find everything from silver-embossed white cards (£1.69 for six), to tear-off pads of invitations (£1.75 for twenty sheets). Branches of Paperchase dotted around the south of England sell a lively range of designs. W. H. Smith, Ryman and print shops such as KallKwik all have catalogues of designs they can print specially for you.

Bizzie Lizzie make personalized cards for christenings and birth announcements, printing inserts to suit each customer. They have a range of designs incorporating gold or silver lettering on parchment paper. Cards cost £22 for the first twenty and £8 for each consecutive ten. You can have a little ribbon bow for 10p extra for each card. Bizzie Lizzie can be reached on 01342 834126.

Handwritten designs are available from **Jane Alnutt** in black ink on coloured card. Prices range from around 90p each to £1.30. Telephone 01245 359865 for details.

Precious Moments can provide classic personalized designs at £29.95 for twenty-five and £39.95 for fifty. These are often found as inserts in parenting magazines. Telephone 01428 727645 for a catalogue.

Flowers

You can always do these yourself. If you want to provide several arrangements for a number of tables, negotiate with your local florist or a trustworthy market trader to order a wholesale box of flowers for you.

Food

Your budget will probably determine the scale of your hospitality. If you are contemplating using outside caterers always get more than one quote. Ideally, test their food before you commit yourself. All major supermarkets do ranges of party food, either fresh or frozen, and some provide selections. Tesco makes up a choice of fresh party platters on a daily basis; Sainsbury and Marks & Spencer both do special lines of miniature cakes and savouries for parties. Most supermarkets will hold items for you if you alert them a few days in advance. The ranges are often expanded in the run-up to Christmas.

Finger buffets are the easiest way to cater for a lot of people as they require less crockery, staff and flowers than a sit-down meal and everything can be prepared beforehand.

Table decorations

If you want personalized coasters, paper plates, napkin rings, serviettes, cake boxes, sweet boxes, bags and ribbons, contact Celebration Stationery for a catalogue on 01332 349931. Discounts are available on large orders. Seven-inch paper plates cost around £9.95 for fifty and serviettes start at £8.95 for fifty. The Party Place offer a huge variety of mail order partywear (tel. 01733 330023).

The countdown

Twelve to ten weeks ahead:
- Agree the service and confirm the time and venue.
- Book the caterers and facilities if applicable.
- Order any personalized stationery you require and check delivery date.
- Choose godparents and check that they will be available. The role and number of godparents differs, depending on your beliefs. They are usually picked from friends or family to act as your child's mentor and care for her in times of crisis.

Six weeks ahead:
- Send out invitations.
- Decide what your baby should wear.

Two weeks ahead:
- Confirm the ceremony details with the participants.
- Check that the godparents are clear about their role on the day.

One week ahead:
- Start organizing food and drink if you are doing it yourself.
- Arrange for any flowers to be ready on the day or the day before the event.

The day before:
- Write yourself a timetable for the day.

On the day:
- Once the food, drink and decorations are prepared, get yourself ready before attending to the baby.
- Give yourself plenty of time to feed and change the baby before leaving for the ceremony.
- If you have other children, bring a bribe in your handbag (e.g. a favourite food that will not ruin clothes) in case you need to inject some silent best behaviour into your brood.

Buying a Gift for a New Baby

Always ask if there is something specific that the parents would like before sallying forth to the shops: they may be finding it hard to leave the house to go in search of a particular item. If you can do it for them, you will earn gratitude for the thought as well as the gift.

Clothes

Be sure to buy a size or two larger than newborn. Nearly all shoppers enjoy buying baby clothes, so new parents can be inundated with clothes for babies under six months, some of which may never be worn. Go for a larger size and pray that the parents don't forget about it.

Marks & Spencer have launched a wonderful variety of luxurious babywear at fair prices – look for the Petit Bébé range. M&S also sell large shawls for £16. Both Boots and Mothercare also stock clothing suitable for gifts.

If you want baby clothes delivered gift wrapped to home or hospital, Mini Boden mail order (0181 964 2662) has a range of classic clothes. If the recipient does not like your choice he or she can change it for something else in the catalogue.

Unbreakable Crockery

Unbreakable plates, cups etc. are always welcome. Mothercare have a zappy new range of feeding and food-storage items in bright, translucent colours. Boots, Children's World and Sainsbury also carry some cheerful, practical designs.

Bibs

Bibs are always useful. A very few stockists have the Baby Bjorn pelican bib for babies of three months upwards. This is made of very soft plastic with a wide shelf to catch drips. More rigid pelican bibs are not suitable until babies are considerably older.

Co-ordinates

If the wallpaper and soft furnishings in the nursery have come from one store, such as Designers' Guild, Mothercare or the Early Learning Centre, the parents may want some particular items to match. Alternatively, you can just get hold of the appropriate fabric from the same shop and make something yourself, such as a simple drawstring bag for laundry or pyjamas to hang on the back of the door.

Bath Accessories

Mothercare have some fun boxed sets of towels and flannels. Personalized towels are available from Letterbox Presents mail order (01872 580885) starting at £9.99 for a cuddle wrap, a towel suitable for babies up to fifteen months.

Photograph Frames

A Feast of Frames is a wonderful mail-order catalogue which is bound to have a frame to suit your taste and your purse. Their range includes mini baby albums, personalized frames and self-adhesive montage frames. Call 0171 738 9632 to order a catalogue.

Toys See Chapter 18.

Books

Board books, cloth books or waterproof books for the bath make good presents. Most babies love pictures of other babies. Dorling Kindersley publish a huge variety of suitable titles for parents to enjoy with children of all ages.

Music

Cassettes or CDs for the car may be appreciated. The Early Learning Centre, Woolworth and many bookshops offer musical selections for babies.

Personalized Gifts

The Letterbox Presents mail order as above has personalized door plaques (£8.99), mugs (from £6.99), hanging names in fabric (£9.99 plus £2 per letter), teddies with a personalized scarf (£19.99), aprons (from £7.99), towels, watercolours, bags, pom-pom hats, children's furniture, brushes, cushions, tablemats and everything else you could think of.

Eximious (tel. 0171 235 7828 for the shop at 10 West Halkin Street, London, SW1X 8JL, or for details of their mail-order service) has a small upmarket selection including a pewter mug with a handle resembling a nappy pin and personalized children's wooden hangers (£16.50 for three).

Silver

Sterling-silver tooth-fairy boxes (around £30), photograph frames and trinket boxes can be found in jewellers and larger department stores. Harman Brothers supplies a range of such items: telephone them on 0121 554 9391 to find a stockist near you.

A silver-plated tooth-fairy box with the baby's name and birthdate engraved on the top can be supplied by Celebration Books mail order (tel. 01428 727645), price £9.99, as can a silver birth certificate-holder (£29.99) and a pewter keepsake box (4in in diameter) for a baby's birthtag, first tooth and first curl. The top is engraved with storks and a clock personalized with first name, weight, date and time of birth (£22.99).

Dartmoor Silvershoe (tel. 01822 81718) will electroplate

in silver or copper a baby's dummy or shoe. Prices from £19.

The baby can adopt a 'baby' of its own via animal adoption schemes run at most large zoos. Adopting an animal at London Zoo costs from between £20 and £30. Tel. 0171 586 4443 for details.

A case of port is a traditional gift but remember that not every year is vintage – take advice before you buy. 1996 babies may grow up to enjoy some 1991 'end bond', costing around £140–£205 and stored at a cost to you of £5 to £6 per year until delivered, when duty and VAT will be payable. Corney and Barrow (est. 1780) will sell, store and deliver your port (tel. 0171 221 5122).

> **!!!** With all mail-order items, be sure to get a catalogue before placing an order so that you can see what you are buying.

Gifts of Money

See pages 77–85.

Giving a Present on Behalf of the Baby

Doting family members will have a happy reminder of the baby with a Smile Calendar. Choose twelve of your favourite baby pictures and Smile will copy and enlarge them to produce a full-colour calendar. Prices are around £21.95 but the unit price drops, depending on how many you order. Tel. 01483 440944, or write to Smile Calendars, PO Box 365, Guildford, Surrey GU4 8YN.

9 Parents and Carers

Fatherhood

Fathers and the Law

If you are married, you and your partner share responsibility for your child until he is eighteen or is legally adopted. If you are not married, responsibility lies solely with the mother.

If you do not want to be in a position where you support your baby financially but have no say in how your money is spent and you want legal responsibility for your child, send off for Children and Young Persons: The Parental Responsibility Agreement Regulations 1991 (Statutory Instrument 1991 No. 1478), available from HMSO Publications, PO Box 276, London SW8 5DR (tel. 0171 873 9090), enclosing a cheque for £1.05. You can also apply for legal responsibility through the courts, but consult a solicitor in the first instance.

Dealing with Pregnancy

Around 10 per cent of expectant fathers experience genuine sympathetic physical symptoms during their partner's pregnancy. Known as *couvade*, these can range from a distended stomach to contractions.

If you are not one of the unlucky 10 per cent but would like some idea of the joys of pregnancy, your local hospital may be able to lend you an empathy belly. This is a vinyl tummy and bosom that you can strap on to yourself to see how pregnancy feels. The belly is filled with water to simulate the sensation of the foetus moving around and a specially constructed beanbag presses down on the bladder for increased authenticity. If you want your own, they cost £1,066.10 from Health Edco, PO Box 1090, Pulborough, West Sussex RH20 4YY, tel. 01903 745444.

> !!! If you suffer from a chronic medical condition such as high blood pressure, asthma or epilepsy, do not use an empathy belly.

Being Present During Labour

Antenatal classes are good preparation for fathers who want to be present at the birth or whose partners would like them to attend. But just because most fathers attend births, it may not be right for you. Think about it and discuss it with your partner well in advance. If you decide not to be there, be sure to get a thorough run-down on how it went from either the midwife, the obstetrician or the alternative birth partner. This might make it easier for you to understand how the new mother feels.

> **PLUS POINTS**
> * Such an intense experience brings you closer together.
> * Just by being there you can give your partner tremendous emotional support.
>
> **MINUS POINTS**
> * It can be deeply distressing to see someone you love in pain.
> * You may find it difficult to see your partner as your lover for quite a while after you have witnessed her giving birth.

If you decide to be there

If your partner starts screaming for an epidural when she previously said she did not want one in any circumstances, do not contradict her. No one can know in advance what pain is going to be like.

Dr Helen Murphy advises: 'It is better to have an epidural and enjoy the birth than to go through hell and have terrible memories afterwards.'

If your partner starts swearing at you, recognize this as a normal reaction from someone who is in extreme pain and absolutely exhausted. Do not take it personally. Stand by her head, where you can hold her hand and give her emotional support. Many men find it disturbing to see their partner's genital area in a distended and gory condition.

If you decide not to be there

- Ensure that your partner has with her someone else she can trust, such as a sister.
- Make sure that the hospital has made a written note that someone else will be attending in your place.
- Be within easy reach so that you can see and hold your baby as soon as he is born.

Paternal Instinct

It is rare for a new mother to know instinctively how to care for a first baby. She will need help with breastfeeding or to be shown how to hold a bottle so that the baby does not take in too much air. But as mothers are expected to learn quickly, they do. Fathers are not pressurized to perform in the same way, and as a result many feel surplus to requirements. If you know you want to participate in the care of your baby, you must make your feelings known. You cannot expect anyone to read your mind.

If your partner finds it hard to share the baby, explain how important it is for you as a family unit that both parents are involved. Maybe one task could always be yours, perhaps bathing the baby at bedtime or taking him out for a walk.

Helpful organizations

Pippin Groups support expectant and new parents in their changing relationship with each other during pregnancy and their relationship with their baby after the birth. Contact them at Derwood, Todds Green, Stevenage, Herts, SG1 2JE, tel. 01438 748478.

Parent Network, 44–6 Caversham Road, London NW5 2DS, tel. 0171 485 8535, organize education and support groups for improving relationships with children. Fathers are especially welcome. Parent Network has developed a thirteen-week programme of parenting education known as 'Parent-Link'. Participants talk to other group members about the daily stresses of parenting, and learn strategies for handling family conflict in ways that can benefit everyone.

If you feel that you are finding parenting too stressful, call Parentline on 01702 559900, or (Eire) 873 3500.

Further reading

The Uncertain Father by Richard Seel, Gateway, £4.95.
The NCT produce a leaflet entitled *Becoming a Father*, which is available through NCT Maternity Sales, Glasgow, tel. 0141 633 5552.

Single Parenthood

One in five families is headed by a single parent. If you feel panic-stricken or lonely as you contemplate your future, you can call on many organizations who offer both practical and emotional assistance. Some of them are listed below.

Benefits

One in ten single parents manage on income support as it is often more cost-effective than going out to work. Make sure that you claim everything you can. *If in doubt, put in a claim.* You will be told soon enough if you are wrong. If the forms seem unintelligible, the Citizens' Advice Bureau will help you fill them in.

Benefits for which you may be eligible are:
- one-parent benefit;
- child benefit;
- income support;
- family credit;
- housing benefit.

For details see Chapter 3.

Labour

If you are a single pregnant woman, your positive decision to go it alone may discourage friends or family from offering you their help. They may well assume that you will turn them down. But you can ask any adult to be with you during labour. To avoid misunderstandings:
- Be sure that the name of your birth partner is added to your medical notes well in advance.
- Suggest that your birth partner accompanies you to an appropriate antenatal class to be clear about what is expected of him or her.

Helpful organizations

- **Gingerbread**, 35 Wellington Street, London WC2E 7BN, tel. 0171 240 0953; Gingerbread Scotland, Community Central Hall, 304 Maryhill Road, Glasgow G20 7YE, tel. 0141 353 0953; Gingerbread Northern Ireland, 169 University Street, Belfast BT7 HYR, tel. 01232 231417; offers nationwide support and activities for single parents. Their phone line is open from Monday to Friday between 11 a.m. and 2 p.m.
- The **Meet-a-Mum Association**, c/o Briony Hallam, 14 Willis Road, Croydon, Surrey, CR0 2XX, tel: 0181 665 0357,

has nationwide groups and support for mothers of young children.
- The **National Association of Citizens' Advice Bureaux**, tel. 0171 833 2181, will tell you where your local office is if you cannot find it.
- The **National Council For One-Parent Families**, tel. 0171 267 1361, offers free information and advice for single parents, including help with claiming welfare payments and benefits.
- The **Working Mothers' Association**, 77 Holloway Road, London N7 8JZ, has a wide range of information on all aspects of childcare and employment rights for women returning to work.
- The **Federation of Services for Unmarried Parents and Children** (Eire), tel. 496 4155.

Childcare

If you are returning to work you will obviously need to arrange for someone to look after your baby or child. Today's childcare involves expense and compromise, but there are workable solutions. The essential ingredients for successful childcare are:
- Continuity of care.
- A good children-to-carer ratio.
- Fully trained carers.
- You have interviewed the carers to your satisfaction.
- You have checked his or her references.

Childminders

Childminders look after other people's children in their own home and are self-employed. All carers for children under eight years old must be registered with the local authority, who check the childminder's home annually to ensure that standards are maintained. Childminders have to uphold safety procedures and keep records about the children in their care. By law a registered childminder can mind only one child under twelve months old at a time and not more than two under eighteen months. They cost between £50 and £90 per week.

You need someone who:
- you feel you can talk to;
- is enthusiastic and loves children;
- has lots of toys and books around the home and encourages the children to use them;
- has a garden with outdoor toys.

Arrange to visit her home and take your baby with you. See how she treats her. Watch how she treats the other children she looks after. Do they respond to her in a happy, loving way? Also ask if you can talk to a parent of another child in her care. Be wary if the house is extremely tidy – it might be a sign that housework takes precedence over childcare – or if she looks after older children, maybe her own, who need a lot of driving around, or if the television is constantly on.

Finding a childminder

The best way is by word of mouth. Otherwise your local authority social services will hold a register of childminders in your area. You may also be able to find the list in your local library or health centre. Look for advertisements in local newspapers or shop windows.

The National Childminding Association (NCMA) can put you in touch with a local childminder. You can obtain at a cost of £2 their book, *A Parents' Guide to Childminding*. Also available is a factsheet, *A Negotiating Guide for Parents* (75p), which deals with rates of pay. The NCMA can be contacted at 8 Masons Hill, Bromley, Kent BR2 9EY, tel. 0181 464 6164.

Don't feel embarrassed about having to ask lots of questions. A good childminder will welcome the opportunity to show off an efficient set-up and would be surprised if you did not thoroughly examine her before leaving your child in her care.

Questions to ask

- Is she registered and insured (can you see her certificates)?
- What are her charges? Does she charge by the hour or the week?
- Are there any extra charges for food or outings?
- What hours is she willing to work?
- How flexible is she if hours alter at short notice?
- What alternative arrangements exist for when she is sick or on holiday?
- Does she have any pets?
- Does she smoke?
- How many other children does she care for, and how old are they? Does she have a routine with which your baby would have to fit in (for example, other children being dropped off and picked up from school)?
- Can she give examples of food she would give your baby?
- Who else would be at home during the day?
- What first-aid training does she have?
- Is there somewhere quiet for the children to rest?
- How often is the television on?
- Does she intend to take the baby out in her car? If so, where? What seating arrangements are there?
- Does she organize any special activities outside her home?
- Does she structure her time so that each child's needs for one-to-one attention are met?
- What play activities does she see as important?
- How would she discipline a child?

Drawing up a contract

If you are taking on a nanny or a childminder it is essential to draw up a contract to prevent misunderstandings. It should include the following:

- Your name, address and telephone numbers where you can be reached, both at home and at work.
- The childminder's name, address and telephone number.

- Contact details of the social services department where the childminder is registered.
- Name and age of the child to be cared for.
- Name of the parent responsible for paying.
- When payment is expected: daily or weekly, in advance or arrears.
- Rates for overtime, unsociable hours, public holidays and weekends.
- What the childminder will charge when the child stays at home if, for example, she is sick or a parent wants to spend some extra time with her.
- The exact hours the contract covers.
- Charges and arrangements for when the childminder is sick.
- Notice time for holidays taken by child or childminder.
- Notice time needed to terminate the agreement or the fee expected by the childminder if notice is not given.
- Who will provide nappies, food, etc.
- Where the childminder can take the child, e.g., shops or library.
- What special events are organized and who pays for them.
- Whether or not the child can travel in the childminder's car.

PLUS POINTS
* Can offer the flexibility to suit your working pattern.
* Gives your baby the security of a home environment.
* Continuous care from one person.
* Provides an opportunity for your baby to be brought up with other local children.

MINUS POINTS
* If your childminder falls ill you may have a serious problem.
* Similarly, if your baby is ill, the childminder will probably not want her in the house with the other children.
* There may be fewer toys and facilities than in a nursery.
* Your child may not have many opportunities to mix with others outside the childminder's home.

Nurseries

There are many types of nursery and they differ widely in philosophy and atmosphere. Local-authority nurseries tend to give priority to children with disabilities or those who are considered 'in need', which can include the children of single parents. Most nurseries open from 8 a.m. to 5 p.m. five days a week. Not all can take babies. By law, all staff must be trained and there must be at least one member for every three children under the age of two. This kind of nursery is different from a nursery school, which is intended to introduce children over three to formal education.

Full daycare can be very expensive, and this is especially the case with private nurseries, particularly in London. Local community nurseries run by local childcare campaign organizations and special interest groups are often cheaper, but places are usually limited. Prices for private nurseries vary from county to county, across London and even within boroughs, but typical fees are between £80 and £100 per week. Community nurseries start at around £70 per week.

The new voucher system

This is a contribution by voucher from the government to help with nursery education for four-year-olds. Only some counties and a handful of London boroughs will be involved in the voucher system pilot scheme at the time of writing. Contact your local authority education department for more details and to find out whether your borough is participating in the scheme.

Finding a Nursery

For information on private nurseries, contact the National Private Day Nurseries Association, tel. 01455 635556. Nurseries, playgroups and nursery schools must be registered with your local social services department, who keep a list.

Questions to ask

- Does the nursery have a 'key-carer' system whereby one member of staff is responsible for each child?
- Are the children split into groups for supervision? How does it work?
- How does the baby spend his day? Does he get taken out of doors? How much one-to-one attention will he receive?
- Is there space for children to run around inside and out?
- Does the nursery keep records of each child's development?
- What type of foods are served?
- How long has the present staff been employed? Is there a high turnover rate?

What to look for

- Is the atmosphere rigid or relaxed and happy?
- Are the babies left on their own except for feeding and changing?
- Do the babies mix with the older children at all?
- Do the staff seem happy and responsive to the children?
- Is the equipment and building properly cared for?
- Is there an outdoor play area?

PLUS POINTS
* Nurseries are usually open during normal office hours and throughout the school holidays.
* You will not have to make alternative arrangements at short notice as you may have to with a childminder.
* Your child mixes with children of different ages and other adults.
* A range of toys, games and activities is available.
* It is easier for parents to see what goes on all day and state their likes and dislikes.
* Carers are fully trained.

MINUS POINTS
* Rigid opening times can be a problem if you are delayed.
* There may not be a lot of one-to-one attention.

Playgroups

If you are looking for extra assistance with an older child while you concentrate on the new baby, a playgroup may be the answer. Playgroups tend to be run by local community organizations for the two-and-a-half-to-five-year age group, usually on a part-time basis with sessions lasting around three hours. 'Opportunity playgroups' are set up for children with special needs. All playgroups must be registered with your local authority. Prices can vary enormously, but as a guideline the average is £2.70 per session.

Finding a playgroup

You can get a list of local playgroups from social services and some libraries and health centres. The Pre-School Learning alliance (0171 837 5513) can put you in touch with a playgroup near you. Playgroups held on playbuses are organized by the National Playbus Association (tel. 01179 775375).

Questions to ask

In addition to the questions suggested for nurseries, ask the following:
- How many staff are employed and how many children are they expected to care for?
- How many of the staff are trained?
- Are parents encouraged or expected to join in?

PLUS POINTS
* A good way for toddlers to meet others and develop through structured play activities.
* Most groups tend to run morning or afternoon sessions so toddlers can attend at a time that is convenient for you.

MINUS POINTS
* Playgroups usually offer only part-time care.
* Most groups start at around 9 to 9.30 a.m., which may not fit in with your working hours.

Caring for Your Baby in Your Own Home

Over 50 per cent of pre-school children are looked after by relatives, friends and neighbours. This may prove not as reliable as a professional childcare option. To make it work, it is essential that you all agree on the basics, for instance, food, potty training and discipline.

Nannies

A nanny is a carer who looks after your baby in your home. As her employer, you are responsible for the standard of care she offers as well as her contract, tax and national insurance. Professional nannies tend to avoid jobs that involve additional duties not relating to the child, so be very clear on what is expected (a mother's help, on the other hand, will assist with cleaning and other household duties). A trained nanny has an NNEB (Nursery Nurse Examination Board) qualification or equivalent.

A nanny's typical wage is betwen £120 and £200 per week, plus tax and national insurance. Those who live out tend to charge more as they have living expenses to cover.

You will have to screen all applicants yourself. The best way to do this is to ask specific questions over the telephone (for example, details of qualifications and experience, and whether the candidate is a driver or a smoker). If her answers seem satisfactory, ask her to send you a CV. Only then, if it all looks fine, should you invite her for interview.

Someone who interviews well is not necessarily going to be the ideal person for looking after babies. You do not want your child to be the casualty of a nanny's indifference or ineptitude. Invite her to spend a morning with your baby. Watch how she handles him. 'Baby-loving' nannies are easy to spot: they cannot bear to put the baby down. Be very, very careful about references. Always take them up.

If you are employing a live-in nanny, it is worth investing in an extra phone line for her room so that she can answer it herself and pay her own bills. Otherwise you will find that you arrive home from work only to be constantly running to pick up the phone. It is always for her, and your own friends can never get through.

Finding a nanny

You can find a nanny employment agency in the Yellow Pages but these tend to be expensive. London agencies include the Lonsdale (0181 876 0020), the Nanny Service (0171 935 3515) and Kensington Nannies (0171 937 2333), which cover a broad spectrum of nannies and mothers' helps in the London area.

Advertising in the *Lady* (published weekly at 65p) is the cheapest option. It costs £14.74 for the first ten words and £6.70 for every additional five.

The Good Nanny Guide, a Vermilion paperback, is indispensable. It covers everything you need to know about nannies as well as listing loads of reputable agencies and colleges where nannies can be found.

You may be able to find a nanny fresh from one of Britain's private training colleges, such as the Norland (01488 681164), Princess Christian (0161 224 4560) or Chiltern (01734 471 847). The Rangi Ruru Nanny School in New Zealand turns out equally professional individuals, many of whom wish to work in Britain. They can be reached via the London agencies mentioned above.

Drawing up a contract

It should contain the following as a minimum. You may wish to cover additional points.
- Name and address of employer and employee.
- Starting date.
- Probation period, if any.
- Length of stay.

- Notice on both sides.
- Salary (excluding National Insurance and tax, which the employer pays).
- How and when it is paid.
- Sick-pay arrangements.
- Pension (details must appear by law, even if there is no pension with the job, as is the case with most nanny positions).
- Hours of work (you may wish to put 'variable' here if you are employing a nanny for the first time and are not quite sure how your working week will shape up).
- The amount of evening babysitting expected per week or per month.
- Time off (how much per week).
- Associated duties (such as keeping the children's toys, clothes and bedrooms well maintained, clean and tidy).
- House rules (smoking, use of telephone, car, etc.).
- Sackable offences (such as inviting unknown people into the house without the employer's permission, gossiping about employer, neglect of charge).

Tax, Insurance and Nannies

If you employ a nanny, you are legally obliged to keep a proper payroll record and to pay her income tax and National Insurance contributions. This is a time-consuming and potentially fraught exercise. For an annual fee of £120 plus VAT, Nannytax will sort all this out on your behalf. Contact PO Box 988, Brighton BN2 1BY, tel./fax 01273 626256.

If you are concerned that your nanny might have an accident while in your employ, check whether your domestic household policy can be extended free of charge. It may well include employer's liability cover, which covers the cost of a claim against you as an employer from an employee working in your home.

> **PLUS POINTS**
> * You can specify precisely what you want for your baby – what he eats, who he sees.
> * Your baby is brought up in his own familiar environment.
> * Flexible working hours can be agreed.
> * Your baby gets one-to-one attention.
>
> **MINUS POINTS**
> * Expensive.
> * Having a live-in nanny can infringe on your privacy.

Nannyshare

If you want a nanny but cannot afford one, consider sharing someone with another family – a cost-effective way of enjoying the benefits of a nanny. Regular meetings between the two families and the nanny are essential to deal with any problems before they escalate.

You will need to decide how you would envisage this working, as each nannyshare differs, depending on the nanny and the families involved. For example, where will the nanny live – with one family? Or will she live out? Would one home be her base, or would she alternate between the two? Do both families require babysitting, etc.?

Finding a nanny to share

To find the right family to share with, you might try talking to friends, asking your local NCT or health visitor or advertising in your local newsagent. The total cost to be shared will probably be slightly higher than for a nanny looking after one child.

Contracts

For a nannyshare to work, both households should agree on the terms already outlined for a contract between one employer and a nanny, and draw up a contract to cover them. In addition, you will need to stipulate how long the nannyshare will last and what the procedure will be if one family likes the nanny and the other does not. Consider how to jointly share the costs, not forgetting hidden extras such as wear and tear on your property by another child, extra equipment, higher insurance premiums on your car so that the nanny can drive the children around, and how to cope if your nanny is sick.

PLUS POINT
* Costs are pooled.

MINUS POINT
* Equipment and wear-and-tear costs can be high.

Mother's Help

A mother's help tends to have no qualifications but may undertake light cleaning work and cooking in addition to childcare. Traditionally, a mother's help would assist a mother staying at home around the house, but nowadays they are often left in sole charge. If you are going to leave your baby with someone who has no training, you might consider sending them on a first-aid course.

Many people rave about mothers' helps from Australia and New Zealand. Although they tend not to stay long, Antipodean girls tend to be treasured members of the household due to their tremendous energy and enthusiasm.

Although there are a number of agencies dealing direct with Australia, you could advertise in *TNT*, the free publication for Australians and New Zealanders living in London (tel. 0171 937 3985).

Again, you must check all references, even if it involves expensive long-distance phone calls.

Both the *Lady* and nanny agencies also list mothers' helps. Wages are around £90 to £130 per week.

Babysitting

When it comes to babysitting, most teenagers are happy to work for pocket money. There are no laws governing babysitting, but bear in mind that a teenager under sixteen cannot be held legally responsible for anything that happens to a child in his or her care. Always leave a contact number and be back on time. Give details of any comforters your baby uses, for example a blanket or teddy. You should pay £2 to £5 per hour, depending on the sitter's age and experience, and whether or not he or she does additional tasks such as housework.

Make it clear beforehand:
- How much you will pay them.
- What they can take from the fridge.
- What you expect of them. Can they change a nappy?
- What to do in an emergency.
- Whether they can have friends or a boyfriend or girlfriend there in your absence.
- What the arrangements are for getting them home (unless they stay overnight).
- Whether they can use the telephone.

Crèches

Crèches are temporary childcare facilities that are operated by employers, at specific events or in public places such as shopping centres. Staff are not necessarily trained. Only leave your child if you feel confident about both the standard of care and security arrangements. They usually cost £2 to £2.50 an hour.

Au Pairs

An au pair comes from overseas and expects to be treated as an equal in your family. Unlike a nanny, her prime concern is to learn English. Looking after your baby or child provides the means to do this. An au pair is therefore ideal if you want an extra pair of hands, but unsuitable as a full-time carer. However, the term 'au pair plus' is sometimes used to describe an au pair who, by arrangement with her employer, works extra hours. Wages depend on hours worked, but a local agency will give you a rough idea of what you should expect to pay. An au pair should not work more than thirty hours a week and should receive a minimum of £36 a week.

PLUS POINT
* Minimal costs.

MINUS POINTS
* An au pair is likely to have a poor command of English, which may have serious implications for a child's development.
* She is unlikely to have any training in childcare.
* She does not work more than thirty hours a week and must have one work-free day.

Temporary Help with a New Infant

Contact your local further education college and find out if they run a nursery-nurse training course. As students on the course have to have practical experience, they will probably be delighted to help out with a new baby or twins. This service is usually free and you do get a chance to interview prospective helpers before taking them on. It is not advisable to leave the babies alone with an inexperienced carer, but at least you will have an extra pair of hands.

Maternity Nurses

A maternity nurse is a trained nanny who specializes in the care of newborn babies. It depends on the individual how much care she also offers to the new mother. If it is a 'live-in' position, she will be on duty twenty-four hours a day except for her weekly day off.

Maternity nurses are expensive but are particularly worthwhile if you are expecting more than one baby. You might find a maternity nurse with experience of twins. All hours and terms are subject to negotiation, but expect to pay £250 plus per week. Jobs usually last between two and six weeks.

A good maternity nurse is like gold dust, so start looking when you are around four months' pregnant. Advertise in the *Lady* or register with as many agencies as you feel you can cope with.

Good maternity nurses are often found by word of mouth, so if you are expecting more than one baby, ask at your twins club. There may be a member who can recommend a particular maternity nurse with whom you can deal direct. This will save you paying agency fees.

If you unexpectedly give birth and need a maternity nurse immediately, do give the agencies a ring – there may be somebody somewhere who is free.

Always take up references yourself – do not rely on the agency to do so.

Helpful organizations

Daycare Trust/National Childcare Campaign, 4 Wild Court, London WC2B 4AU, tel. 0171 405 5617, is a charity which gives advice on setting up childcare provisions for a day or community nursery. They also give parents information and contact numbers within their local boroughs.

The **Pre-School Learning Alliance** (formerly the PPA, the Pre-School Playgroups Association), on 0171 837 5513, runs a similar scheme. They have a helpline for parents and carers looking for childcare and advice. They will put you in contact with a fieldworker in your area who has details of nurseries registered with them.

Choices in Childcare, Holly Building, Holly Street, Sheffield S1 2GT, tel. 0114 276 6881, keeps records of local childcare. The central office can put you in touch with the nearest childcare information service to you, where you can talk to somebody about the options available in your area. There are about thirty-five such services in the UK at present holding up-to-date information tailored to parents' needs on all childcare registered with social services – that is, nurseries, childminders and playgroups. For example, if you already have a list of childminders, the local childcare information service will hold specific details about them, such as any pets they might keep, whether they smoke, will do school runs and so on.

This service will also tell you what is going on near you and provide 'out and about' information.

Gingerbread, 16–17 Clerkenwell Close, London EC1R 0AA, tel. 0171 336 8183, offers help and advice on childcare to single parents. They recommend a book called *Free to Work*, written in conjunction with Sainsbury.

The **National Playbus Association**, 93 Whitby Road, Brislington, Bristol, Avon BS4 3QF, tel. 0117 977 5375, can inform you of the nearest association to you and also advise on setting up a playbus. **Parents at Work**, 77 Holloway Road, London N7 8JZ, tel. 0171 628 3578, produce the *Working Parents' Handbook* (£5.50) which provides information on nurseries, nannies, the pros and cons and how to go about arranging childcare.

Other useful organizations are the **National Childminding Association**, 8 Masons Hill, Bromley, Kent BR2 9EY, tel. 0181 464 6164; the **National Private Day Nurseries Association**, Dennis House, Hawley Road, Hinckley, LE10 0PR, tel. 01455 635556; the **Pre-School Learning Alliance**, 69 King's Cross Road, London WC1X 9LL (helpline: 0171 837 5513); the **Irish Pre-School and Playgroup Association**, tel. 671 9245.

PART FOUR
GETTING TO THE BOTTOM OF IT

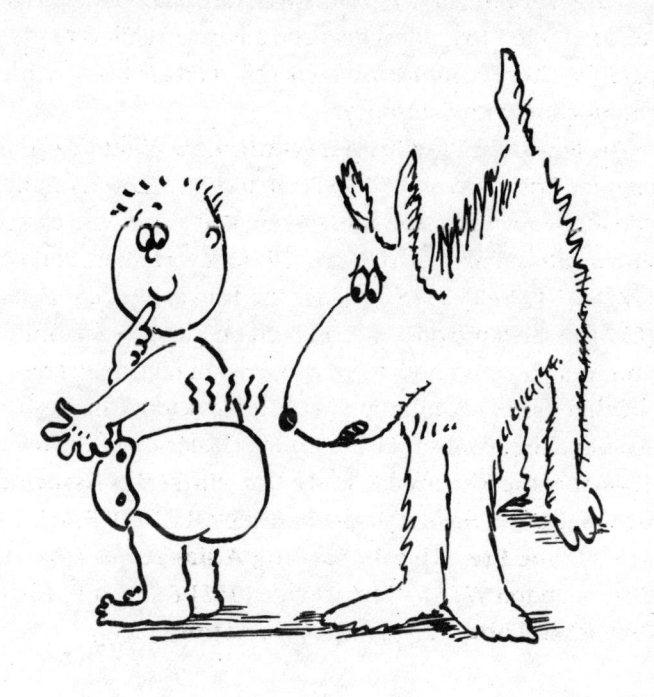

10   Changing Your Baby

Nappies

A baby uses over 2,000 nappies in her first year. When you think that a packet of fifty disposables retails at around £5.50, nappies become a major financial consideration.

Disposables v. reusables

There is no doubt that disposables are extremely convenient, but there are ideological as well as financial reasons to choose reusables, as we saw in Chapter 6.

- You will save nearly £600 over the time your baby is in nappies and still have nappies that you can use for your next baby.
- Disposables generate waste of eight tons per hour in Britain alone.

Which? examined green arguments for and against disposable nappies and suggested that, although disposable nappies create waste, the increased need for electricity to wash reusables was also ecologically damaging (electricity is partially produced by fossil fuels containing pollutants which contribute to global warming).

The most ecologically sound alternative might be to opt for reusable nappies and have them washed by a nappy service. They wash so many nappies at once that they use less water and energy than a number of individuals washing their own nappies separately at home. The service supplies a deodorized nappy pail and hires out a set of nappies exclusively for your use. Each week the soiled nappies are collected and replaced with a laundered supply. This service costs £6 or £7 a week. Sometimes you have to buy your own nappy covers. With a nappy service:

- If you find you do not like reusables you can just stop: check whether your local nappy service requires you to sign up for a specific number of weeks.
- You do not have a hefty outlay for a set of reusables (around £80).
- Overall, it may work out cheaper than disposables.

To find a service near you, telephone the National Association of Nappy Services (NANS) on 0121 693 4949.

Disposable Nappies

Disposable nappies are used by 75 per cent of new mothers. Made of paper products and plastic, they have elasticated legs which stop leaks without constricting the baby's thighs. Reusable tapes at the waist allow you to check if the nappy is wet and seal it again. (In practice, you will find it easier to look down a leg-hole.) Some nappies have wetness indicators. The reusable tapes can also hold a dirty nappy tightly rolled up prior to disposal. Girls' nappies have more padding in the middle while the boys' variety have more at the front.

Always keep a small roll of Sellotape handy when changing a disposable nappy: if you get any powder, lotion or cream on the tapes, they will not stick.

You can use 'nappy sacks' or old plastic carrier bags for soiled disposables, or buy a nappy pail – a plastic bin with a tight-fitting lid to contain smells. Another option is the Sangenic, a nappy-disposal system that compresses and twists up to three days' dirty nappies in thin plastic casing so that they look like a string of sausages which you then put into the dustbin. It costs £19.99 from large chemists and nursery retailers.

Buying Disposables

It is essential to buy the right size: a proper fit minimizes the possibility of leakage, which occurs with both nappies that are either too big and loose, or those that are too small. You should be able to slip one finger under the waistband.

Buying in bulk is a false economy. A baby's growth rate is so fast that you cannot predict when she'll shoot out of one size and be ready for another.

Get the cheapest nappies for your baby's first two weeks. You will change her so many times and there is so little in them that a super-de luxe model is a waste of money.

*** Star buys ***

Nappy prices are extremely variable and special discounts are often available. The prices given here are intended as a guide only.

Testers gave the following the seal of approval:

For a newborn in hospital, Boots Ultra (£3.75 for twenty-four).

Pampers, the Calvin Klein of nappies, seem to fit all shapes and sizes of bottoms (£6.25 for forty for 9 to 20lb baby).

Sainsbury's Performers (£5.59 for fifty) performed just as well.

These were closely followed by Tesco Ultra Dry Advances (£5.59).

Nappy tapes

If you want to help BLISS, the charity that supports babies who need special care, buy a pack of nappy tapes for 99p. These sticky strips allow you to reseal an unsticky nappy tab. They should be available from most major retailers by the end of 1996.

Reusables (Washable Nappies)

You have the choice of a basic terry-towel square or a shaped fabric nappy that looks like a disposable.

Shaped Nappies

These are usually a good fit due to the elasticated waist and legs, and are easy to put on with no folding or fiddling. Some have integral waterproofing, obviating the need for plastic pants. But they can take up to eight hours to dry. Some types depend on safety pins to stay together. If the pinning drives you mad, sew on Velcro tabs for an extremely snug fit.

Terries

These dry quickly, and are half the price of shaped nappies. You need fewer terries than shaped nappies. Nappi Nippas (see Star Buy below) are invaluable.

Soaking dirty nappies in sanitizing fluid removes stains and saves having to boil them. (You can make your own using one cup of vinegar to three gallons of water.) Rinse nappies before putting them in the washing machine – sanitizing fluid can affect the door seal. If you put nappies out to dry on a clothes horse they can become stiff. Line-drying makes them soft, otherwise a tumble drier is fine. Fabric conditioners will soften terries, but they might cause an allergic reaction. If so, switch to a suitable hypoallergenic brand.

★★★ Star buys ★★★

Nappi Nippas, plastic fasteners for terry nappies, are much easier and less worrying to use than safety pins. They cost £1.49 for one or £2.97 for three, plus 50p postage and packing, from Nappi Nippas, PO Box 35, Penzance, Cornwall TR18 4YE, or pick them up in John Lewis.

Here are some brands of reusable nappies and stockists.

The **Earthwise Baby** catalogue features a large range of reusable nappies including the 'snap-to-fit' type that last for the entire nappy-wearing time. A good, user-friendly economical buy – one size fits all – you simply adjust the poppers to fit the size of the baby – though they can be loose and bulky on smaller babies. You may also wish to buy Warren Featherbone Nylon Snap Pants to go over them at £3.50 a pair. Order the catalogue from Earthwise Baby, PO Box 1708, Aspley Guise, Milton Keynes MK17 8YA, tel. 01908 585769, fax 01908 585761.

Firstborn, 32 Bloomfield Avenue, Bear Flat, Bath, Avon, tel. 01225 422586.

Bambino Mio, 44 Montgomery Crescent, Bolbeck Park, Milton Keynes MK15 8PR, tel: 01908 240484. Mail order only.

Bumkins from **Nature's Baby**, PO Box 2995, London NW2 1DW, tel. 0181 905 5661.

Kooshies from **PHP**, 12 Thornton Place, London W1H 1FL, tel. 0171 637 1020 or 495 6860. Some testers hated them because of the limited elastic round the legs. Others adored them so much, they said it was enough to convert them from disposables to reusables. They cost £6.50 to £8, depending on size.

Indisposables, 131 Milner Road, Brighton, East Sussex BN2 4BR, tel. 01273 688212.

Zippidys and **Fluffies Overnaps**, **Harlequin Fluffies**, PO Box 534, Seaford, East Sussex, tel. 01323 895730.

The **Green Store**, 9 Green Street, Bath BA1 2JY, tel. 01255 427155.

Mikey Diapers, shaped nappies by mail order (01737 765723). Universally liked, but tend to come up on the small side. The price per nappy is £4 to £5.50, depending on size.

The **Great British Nappy**, PO Box 1, Whimple, Devon EX5 2YY, tel. 01404 822990.

Schmidt Natural Clothing, 155 Tuffley Lane, Gloucester GL4 0NZ, tel. 01452 416016.

Zorbit terries, from independent retailers, are wonderfully soft. Their effectiveness is totally dependent on the person who puts them on. Use Nappi Nippas instead of safety pins.

Cottontails, shaped nappies by mail order from J. R. Productions, 60 Swan Street, Sileby, Leicestershire LE12, tel. 01509 816787. Comfortable and easy to use. They cost £8.99 for two.

Mothercare non-disposables. You may have to grapple with the pin, but these are good-shaped nappies at £15.99 for ten. They fit well, as do the plastic pants (£8.50).

Home delivery

Nappies are extremely bulky to shop for, so the free home delivery service offered by the following is very useful.
- Boots (0800 622 525).
- John Lewis stores.
- Nappy Express, in the London area (0181 361 4040).

> !!! Ensure that anyone who changes nappies in your home has had a polio booster, since you can contract polio from the faeces of a recently vaccinated baby. Always wash your hands thoroughly after a nappy change.

Nappies for swimming

For un-potty-trained babies and toddlers, swimming nappies (Swimsuit Diapers) prevent embarrassing moments in the swimming pool. They cost around £10.50 from Bright Start mail order (0171 483 3929). Also from Kooshies at £6.50, tel. 0171 637 1020.

Nappy Changes

The safest place to change your baby is on the floor. If she sleeps upstairs, you may find it useful to get a changing mat with a raised edge (£6 to £7) to keep downstairs for quick changes. If you buy a changing table, look for one with a cupboard rather than drawers, which can be too shallow to be of practical use.

Baby Wipes

Wipes that come in square boxes are easier to take out one at a time. Some wipes are impregnated with lotion, such as Tesco's, and these double as good make-up removers.

Most people go by which perfume they like the best. Baby Fresh with Ultra Guard Skin Protectant, Tesco's, Sainsbury's, Boots, Waitrose, Baby Wet Ones and Pampers wipes all come in sensible boxes. It is worth buying a Baby Fresh travel pack (59p from Boots, Children's World and independent chemists) to keep in your changing bag and refill as necessary. Boots also do boxes of individually sealed wipes which are ideal for travelling.

Muslin Squares

If you are wondering whether to 'pass' on buying muslin squares, which are traditionally for nappies, this piece by April Chalklin may convince you otherwise.

> Have you ever stood, in all your pregnant glory, in Mothercare, puzzling over the varied, and often incomprehensible paraphernalia of parenthood? Do 'envelope necks' and 'nipple shields' sound like plumber's equipment to you? Do you wake up in a cold sweat in the wee hours wondering what it's all for? Wonder no more, for we shall now impart to you the Great Knowledge, the Indispensable. We bring unto you . . . twenty uses for a muslin square:
> 1. Puke Rag.
> 2. Dribble Blotter.
> 3. Emergency Nappy.

4. Changing Mat.
5. Head Cushion (folded several times).
6. Car Sunshade (when trapped in the window as you roll it up).
7. Sun Hat (for knotted-hanky fans).
8. Back Saver (roll it up into a sausage shape to take the corner out of buggies, chairs etc., so that tinies are lying almost flat).
9. Toy (this has endless possibilities: it can be waved about, used to play peek-a-boo, chewed, scrumpled and thrown).
10. Bib.
11. Comforter (especially if previously used as 1.).
12. Temporary Breast Pad (while you run around trying to find real ones – very sexy).
13. Temporary Play Mat (when visiting friends).
14. Swaddling Sheet.
15. Carrycot Bottom Sheet.
16. Wee Shield (place over newborn boys' nether regions during nappy change, it prevents them from piddling right in your eye).
17. Cloth Nappy Absorbency Booster Pad.
18. Stork Bag (for midwives only, when weighing baby on home visit).
19. Gag (roll it up and bite on it when having that first postpartum pee).
20. Vaporizer (sprinkle with menthol oil, hang up near cot during the cold season).

You can boil them, you can bleach them, you can (if you're loony) iron them. The quintessential piece of baby gear – stick them on your 'things to buy' list.

The above is reproduced with the kind permission of April Chalklin and Karen Liebreich, editor of the Notting Hill and District Newsletter, which first published it.

Changing Bags

Most changing bags fall to bits. This is not because they are badly made, but because they are subjected to such hard wear. They are crammed with bottles and nappies and then left to dangle from prams; they get hurled into the boot of the car, zipped open in a panic, soaked by leaky bottles and suffer numerous inspections from junior members of the household.

Many 'old-hand' mothers do not see the point of a changing bag. Instead:
- If you already have a small sports bag with a zipped waterproof compartment, use that. Nylon rucksacks by Headstart at £8.25, from Argos and sports shops.
- Keep a bag with nappies, clothes and a towel or mat in the car. (The mat is only necessary if you like putting your baby on the floor instead of keeping him in his car seat.)
- The Klippan Carrytot Royal car seat has a special compartment for paraphernalia.
- Keep a folded sleepsuit, spare nappies and a travel pack of wipes under the pram mattress at the baby's feet-end. Feeds are then the only item you need to prepare freshly for each trip out. These can be kept in small insulated bags available from Boots and Mothercare and transported in your handbag.

Buying a changing bag

You may wish to buy a changing bag that co-ordinates with your pram or buggy. Co-ordinates are offered by most major manufacturers. Look for a bag which:
- fits in your pram shopping tray;
- is completely waterproof inside;
- has at least three pockets;
- fastens with a zip – velcro can prove insecure;
- contains a changing mat.

There are four basic designs available.

- The standard shoulder-bag model, large and rectangular.
- The backpack.
- The 'you'd knever know it's a changing bag' changing bag. Looks like a fashion item.
- The bum bag. A small bag for essentials, excluding a bottle and a changing mat.

★★★ Star buys ★★★

(Excluding models that come with prams.)
The Boots Abstract changing bag is a 'standard shoulder bag'. It includes PVC changing mat, wash bag, feeding bag and a wipe-clean bib for £22.99.

The JoJo Maman quilted changing bag, £26.99, is a Chanel-type disguise for nappies and bottles.

The Caboodle bum bag, £9.99, is very compact and can hold a bottle and a nappy. A changing mat is included in the price but you may wish to store it separately.

Keep an eye out in Marks & Spencer – you may be lucky and find that they have a small supply of changing bags. They are consistently excellent but thin on the ground.

PART FIVE
BATHTIME

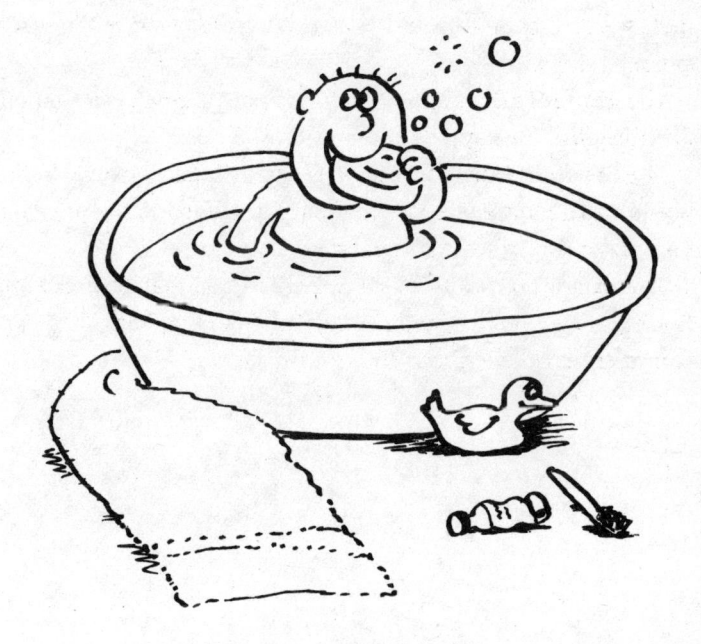

11   In the Bathroom

Many new mothers have visions of their expected baby as a permanently bathed, sweet-smelling little bundle, gently misted with talcum powder. If some of the larger retailers are to be believed, you need a vast array of lotions, potions and equipment to achieve this. Don't be fooled.

Baby Baths

You do not need a baby bath. Buy one only if you have a bad back and need to stand while washing the baby (see changing units, pages 213–14). They do, however, make great sledges.

If you do have to buy a bath, and you have the space to store it when not in use, the Eezi-Bath is recommended. It fits on to the proper bath, you fill it from the taps and the water empties directly into the bath afterwards. It does not fit all baths, so measure yours first and check the baby bath before you unwrap it. The Eezi-Bath is stocked by John Lewis and independent retailers.

Eezi also produce a sponge support for £5.99 (available at Mothercare), which can be used in a larger bath. It is particularly useful if you are attempting to bathe two babies at once. Later on you can cut it up for sponge painting. If your older baby really dislikes water, you can buy him a bath ring, supported by legs that have suction pads to hold it to the base of the bath. The baby goes inside the ring, which reaches his waist, allowing him to sit up in the bath with his face away from the water. But beware – however safe this sounds, fatal accidents can still occur. Babies should never be left in a bath unattended in any circumstances.

Look out for the Fisher Price Stay'n'Play bath ring (£16), which has particularly good suction.

Bath Thermometers

You do not need a bath thermometer, either, if you take the following steps:
- Put cold water into the bath first and then add hot until it is warm enough.
- Swish the water around vigorously so that the heat is evenly spread.
- Test the temperature with your elbow.
- Turn down the thermostat so that the water coming out of the taps is not too hot. (Turning down your thermostat one degree can cut heating bills by 10 per cent and reducing the temperature of your bathwater from scalding to 60 degrees C will save up to £20 a year.)

If you would still feel happier with some sort of thermometer, you can buy one from the Early Learning Centre (£2.99) or, if someone wants to spend some money on the baby, you might ask for the Tubby Elephant set from Baby Basics mail order (01703 234949), price £24. This includes a bath-tap protector and a non-slip bath mat that changes colour when the water is too hot. The Tub Team drain cover is meant to prevent children from hitting their heads against the drain release valve.

> **!!!** Never leave your baby alone in the bath for a second. If you have to turn away, take him out of the bath.

Baby Toiletries

Soap and Baby Bubble Bath

Your baby does not need soap. It can make her skin dry and additives can cause rashes. It is also difficult to hold a slippery, soapy baby.

Your baby does not need liquid baby bath, either. However, she might like playing with the bubbles and you may like the perfume. Johnson & Johnson, Tesco and Boots are among the many manufacturers offering these popular products.

If your baby has dry skin, a few drops of olive oil in the bath can help. Almond oil from pharmacists' counters is a good all-round baby moisturizer that does not make the skin greasy. Your doctor may recommend Oilatum (£4.85 for 250ml) if your baby persistently suffers from dry skin.

You do not need talcum powder, but the smell is wonderful. Traditional nannies still coat their charges in the stuff but many experts worry that too much powder can get into a baby's airways. If you are going to use it, be sure that you have properly dried the baby first.

Cotton buds are useful for fiddly cleaning, but be very careful not to push one into an ear or up a nose. Best value is Boots – 99p for a bag of 250.

Sponges and Flannels

Yet another item you do not need. If you want to use something other than your hands, cotton wool is more hygienic. The best cotton wool for this purpose is Boots' cotton-wool pads (£1.49 for fifty or £2.25 for a hundred). They are flat and embossed to ensure that no fibres are left on the skin after washing or cleaning.

Toothbrush and Toothpaste

Start cleaning your baby's teeth as soon as they appear. A diamond-headed toothbrush such as Colgate's My First Colgate is recommended: its shape allows you to get right to the back of the baby's mouth. It also has a dot on the bristles to show you how much toothpaste to use. Always ensure that your children use a toothpaste that is specifically for children: the content is more appropriate for the care of milk teeth. Maclean's toothpaste for milk teeth (£1.05 for 50ml) is sugar-free and has the correct fluoride level.

Teething Gel

Recommended brands include Dentinox (£1.49 for 10g), which is suitable for use from birth, and Bonjela (£1.99 for 15g) for use from four months. Try giving your baby a piece of cold cucumber to gnaw on. If you take out the seeds in the centre, you can slip a small chunk over her thumb or finger. Never leave a baby alone with food as she may choke.

Child-friendly dentists

If you want a child-friendly dentist when your child's teeth come through, contact the Smile Line, on 0151 230 0240, or write to 17–19 Deysbrook Lane, West Derby, Liverpool L12 8RE, for details of your nearest Mini Molar Club. This is a free club that encourages children to look after their teeth. They have stickers, comics, badges and a membership card.

Fresh from France are Tartine et Chocolat baby perfumes, available at Givenchy counters in perfumery departments. Soap costs £8.75 and Baby Eau de Toilette £17.50.

The Bathroom Cabinet

First Aid

The following list of essentials was prepared with the help of experts at Boots.
- Crêpe bandages.
- Plasters in a variety of shapes and sizes.
- Sterile gauze.
- Sterile dressings, including an eye pad.
- Safety pins and scissors.
- Micropore surgical tape (this is hypoallergenic).
- Tweezers.
- Savlon children's antiseptic (the children's version stings less than the adults').
- Calamine lotion for sore, sunburned skin and rashes.

★★★ Star buys ★★★

Boots first-aid kit (£8.99) is ideal for keeping in the car or the kitchen. It contains a little leaflet explaining what to do in the most common emergencies.

Thermometers

A forehead strip thermometer gives you a fair indication of temperature and is easy to use: you simply hold it against your baby's forehead for around fifteen seconds, and colour changes indicate the temperature. Buy Robinson Feverscan (£2.59), Boots Feverscan (£2.59) or Tommee Tippee Forehead (£2.49).

Electronic digital thermometers are very accurate, usually to within 0.1 of a degree. They take longer to use – three minutes or more – and are more expensive.

★★★ Star buys ★★★

The First Years underarm (£7.99).

Nappy-Rash Preparations

Most people find Sudocrem (£3.99 for 250g) or zinc and castor-oil cream (99p for 125g) work well. If these have no effect, ask the pharmacist to make up a mixture of Lasser's paste with the same amount of Vaseline (cost around £1) or try coating your baby's bottom with egg white.

Cold Remedies

It is common practice in many European countries to extract mucus from a baby's bunged-up nose with a special extractor such as NUK's nasal decongester (£2.95 from chemists). However, a British pharmacist may suggest saline drops (£1 to £2) and Karvol capsules (£1.75 for ten).

Cradle Cap Preparations

Cradle cap is when the skin on a baby's scalp becomes greasy and crusty. Look out for Detinox cradle cap shampoo (£1.99 a bottle) and Boots cradle cap cream (£1.09 for 25g).

Gripe Waters

Many babies suffer with colic during their first months – you might as well have a bottle of gripe water at the ready. Do not expect it to work at once, though an improvement should be seen over a number of days. Infacol is £2.79. Try Chamomilia for a more instant effect. This comes in the form of drops which calm the baby as well as dealing with colic (£3.25 for 25ml at chemists and some health-food stores).

Pain Relief

After three months, it is possible to administer junior paracetamol-based liquids such as Calpol or Boots Pain Relief syrup.

PART SIX
THE NURSERY

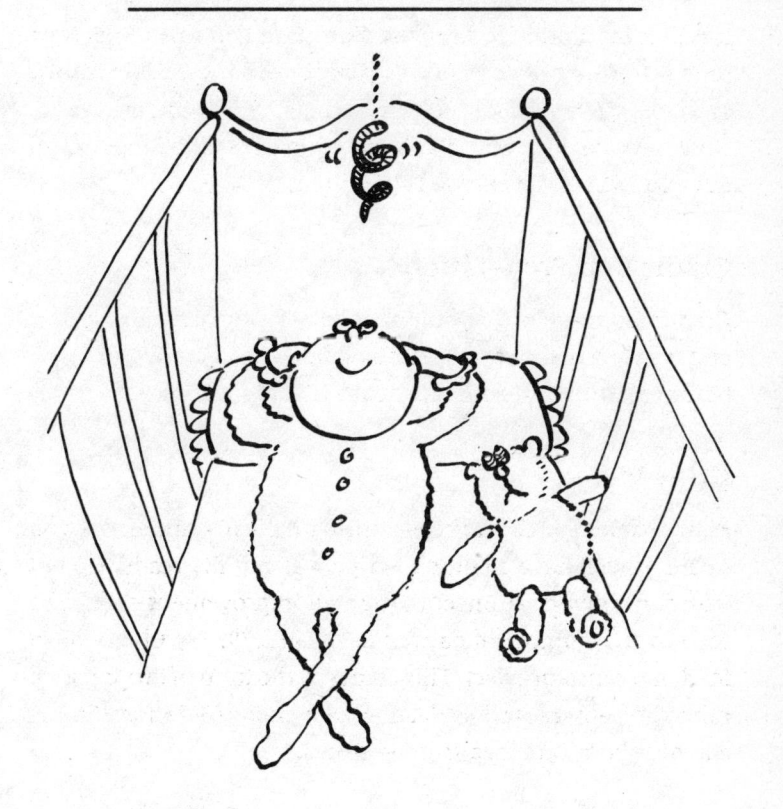

12   Preparing the Nursery

Decorating a Nursery

Bear in mind that your nursery needs to be:
- a peaceful room for sleeping in;
- comfortable to feed and change a baby in;
- a place to store your baby's clothes, toys and equipment.

> !!! Paint your nursery at least a month before the baby moves in so that paint fumes have time to disperse.

Nursery Interior Designers

People who specialize in interior design for nurseries often advertise in the back of parenting magazines. If you want your child to 'enter a different world', contact Harrods interior-design service on 0171 730 1234 ext. 2933.

If you are decorating the nursery without knowing the sex of your baby, Harrods suggests one of the following:
- A neutral colour scheme based on cream or green.
- A duel-sex scheme in yellow and white.
- A white and primary mix.
- Putting up a wallpaper border after the birth to 'prettify' or 'masculinize' the room as appropriate. These are suitable for use with painted walls as well as wallpapers. Remember, however, that the room will need to be hard-wearing.

Paints

For a list of environmentally friendly paint, see page 221. You can buy Plasti-Kote spray paint in aerosol form to use on children's toys, radiators, wrought iron, cane and wicker, wood and plastics. For details, brochure and stockists telephone 01223 836400.

International Paint's toy paint, Japlac and primers are £3.19 for 125ml and £4.69 for 250ml tins. Japlac also come as an aerosol. These paints meet the requirements of the European Toy Safety standards EN71 Part III 1988 and BS5665 Part II 1989. For local stockists call 01703 226722.

ICI Paints says that oil-based coatings are more durable, that is, resistant to bumps and knocks, and will clean up more easily with standard household products. They do, however, take longer to dry and have a very strong smell which will linger for several days after the paint seems dry. ICI Paints recommend leaving the room or items painted for at least a week before allowing a baby to use them.

Water-based coatings dry more quickly and the room can be used very soon after painting, but they are less durable, will mark a little more easily and it will be more difficult to remove marks from the surface.

The choice therefore depends on your circumstances. If a room was last decorated before 1960 it may well have been painted with products containing lead pigments. Even low blood-lead levels can have detrimental effects on young children's intellectual and physical development. During pregnancy, essential elements such as calcium are transferred from the bones of the mother to the baby. This may release accumulated lead. A leaflet entitled *How to Remove Old Lead Paint Safely – A Guide for Painters* is available from the Paintmakers Association (tel. 01372 360660).

Lead-testing kits that will help you test for the presence of lead in the paint film (£12.50 plus VAT) are available from

J. H. Ratcliffe and Co. Paints Ltd (tel. 01704 537999).

The Dulux Advice Line on 01753 550000 can give decorators information on product usage and technical advice.

Decorative Effects

Stencils

The Stencil Library in Northumberland has a thousand designs for nurseries. Designs and stencil equipment are available by mail order on 01661 844844. The catalogue costs £5, which is refundable against purchases.

The Early Learning Centre sells stencils which co-ordinate with their range of fabrics and wallpapers. A stencil of Edward Bear, for example, size 30.5 × 21cm, costs £4.99.

Larger branches of Boots also stock nursery stencil kits, at £5.99.

Stamps

Although the effect is not as subtle, stamps are easier than stencilling. You simply use a block of wood with a cut-out design dipped into paint to decorate furniture and walls.

Ready-made designs from the English Stamp Company are £11.95 for 4in sizes and £5.95 for 2in. The firm can make up any design you require from a black and white illustration of your chosen image for around £14.95 (4in) and £8.95 (2in). These are available by mail order – call 01929 439117 for details.

John Lewis also carries a selection.

Stickers

Slapsticks, gummed paper stickers of favourite storybook characters which can be stuck to walls, doors, windows and wood (but not vinyl wallpaper, plastic or high-gloss surfaces) are available from Leisurebrands Ltd on 01225 874545.

Murals

Several companies take on commissions. Listings can often be found in the back of glossy magazines such as *House & Gardens* or *World of Interiors*. The best source is word of mouth. Otherwise try your local art college.

Co-ordinates

During your pregnancy there will be at least one big sale season – at Christmas or in the summer. This is the best time to buy wallpaper and fabrics: even a small saving per metre of fabric can make a considerable difference to the overall cost.

Harrods point out that if you want a co-ordinated look, you should resist the temptation to go overboard. Your child will soon grow up, and living in a warren of pale blue bunnies when you are a five-year-old Power Ranger is not good for the image.

Nursery ranges of co-ordinated paper and borders are available from the following companies.

Designers Guild (0171 243 7300) at approximately £16 per metre.

Call 01254 870700 for stockists of **Crown Wallcoverings'** Kids Kapers range. Paper starts at £9.99 a roll and borders from £5.99. **Poppy Limited** (01642 790000) offers an attractive selection of co-ordinated fabrics, wallpapers and borders.

Fabric Ranges

Economy buys can always be jazzed up with a border. Mamas & Papas sell borders, fabrics and curtains to match their duvet covers and Moses baskets. But be very careful that you know what you are ordering: their 1995 catalogue shows curtains in their Bertie and Beattie range with a teddy-bear border that co-ordinates with the pelmet. You have to buy this border separately and sew it on to the curtains yourself.

Ian Mankin – checks, stripes and plain – fabrics starting at

£3.50 per metre. Telephone their mail order service, based in one of their London shops, on 0171 722 0097 for free swatches and quotes. Laura Ashley, Homebase, Texas and MFI all sell a wide range. The Play Away collection – 100 per cent cotton, 120cm wide – starts at £5.99 per metre. Call Material World on 0171 585 0125. It is also available through Ashley World Designs on 0171 259 9677. Boras Cotton (01283 550011) have nursery fabrics at approximately £12 per metre.

Windows and Curtains

Thick and fussy curtaining is not appropriate for babies. Curtaining on poles is pretty, but it lets the light in. Whichever curtains you choose, put up a 'black-out' roller blind as well, behind the nursery curtains. Always pull this down at night to regulate your baby's sleep patterns.

Nursery characters to put on the end of curtain poles are available from Hang Ups accessories. Prices start at £28 for a pair of hand-painted characters. They also sell curtain poles (£5.80 per foot, 1.5in wide). Telephone 01285 831771 for details.

Lighting

Try to decide on lighting before you decorate the room. Look out for lampshades which co-ordinate with your chosen paints or wallpapers – the Mothercare ones usually match well – or make a 'mop' lightshade yourself using left-over fabric. Frames are available from A. & J. Lampshades on 0181 648 6776.

You will need dim lighting for night feeds and brighter lighting for changing nappies. Dimmer switches can be used to to lower or increase the central light as needed. Wall lights and spotlights can be fixed to illuminate specific areas of the room.

Bedside lights or nightlights can give security to children who dislike the dark. Battery-operated nightlight toys such as the Tomy Lullaby Lightshow are very popular and safe to use.

Heaters

If your baby's room is very cold, you can fit a thermostatic control valve on the radiator. These cost around £8 from a DIY shop or your plumber.

Stand-alone heaters – fan heaters, paraffin heaters, fires and electric-bar heaters – all pose a threat to your baby's safety. The one to buy is an electric oil-filled radiator. These are thin and relatively unobtrusive. Glen oil-filled radiators are available from Argos, starting at £34.50. You set a thermostat so that the heater clicks off when it reaches the required temperature. Look for a BEAB safety mark – models carrying this cut out automatically if they fall over, and come with wall clips or feet.

> !!! Heaters and babies are a dangerous combination.

- Never allow your baby to crawl on the floor while the heater is on.
- Check that the heater is never set so high that it could burn you or your baby.
- Fireguards must be fitted to the wall to cover electric-bar heaters, fires or paraffin heaters.
- Never place any heater close to the cot.
- Flexes should be kept tidy and short to minimize trailing cables.

Flooring

Avoid rugs, which can be dangerous. Rush matting is abrasive and not particularly long-lasting.

Flip-Flop puzzle mats are interlocking squares which are portable, soundproof, shock-absorbent, and can be used both indoors and outdoors. They are waterproof, childproof and durable and cost from as little as £8.95 to £117.95 for the largest mat. Telephone Sue Fortune on 0191 456 9030 for a colour brochure and stockists.

Harrods suggest, if the nursery is large enough, that you create separate areas by changing the floor finish. A hard-wearing finish such as lino or woodbock can be used for play areas, while a carpeted section is suitable for reading, sleeping, etc.

Nursery Furniture

If you are starting from scratch, Harrods suggest that you:
- select nursery furniture that is readily available so that you can add to it at a later date;
- create more storage space than you think you need.

Nursing Chairs

As so much time during your baby's early months is spent feeding him, it is essential that you are comfortable while you are doing it. John Lewis stocks a specifically designed nursing chair for £325, the Glide R Motion by Dutalier. If you love this chair but would prefer a different fabric, The Baby's Room, 11 Tunsgate, Guildford GU1 3QT, tel. 01483 578984, can supply a full range.

Although you do not need to buy a special nursing chair, you will need a chair with low arms, and firm back support. The Poang from Ikea, which has an exposed beech frame supporting a fabric seat, is ideal for feeding a baby. Prices start at £125, and the top-of-the-range model, in tan buffalo leather, costs £249. Call 0181 208 5600 for your nearest branch.

Changing Units

Changing units are not ideal – one of the most common accidents among babies is rolling or sliding off a changing table.

Do not let go of your baby, or, if you have to, stand in a way that prevents him from rolling off. Many mothers use a waist-high chest of drawers or a table as bending down punishes their backs. This can also be dangerous. You could make a high-sided tray to stand on a chest of drawers but it must be secure. Attach the chest of drawers and the tray to the wall using brackets.

To be 100 per cent safe, change your baby on a changing mat on the floor. The storage provided by a purpose-built unit is not essential: for easily accessible storage for your baby's nappies and lotions, use a vegetable rack. It is cheap and you can see at a glance what you want. If you want to keep all your baby items out ready to use but think it looks messy, cover old formula-milk tins and baby wipe boxes with left-over nursery wallpaper for a co-ordinated look.

If you do choose a purpose-built changing unit, one with a baby bath might be an idea. Otherwise, look for:
- Good stability.
- High sides.
- One that will look good as a chest of drawers or cupboard when you no longer need to change nappies.
- Changing units with cupboards, which tend to be more useful than drawers as these can be rather shallow.

Wardrobes

Baby clothes are so tiny that if you are short of space a wardrobe with standard hanging space is not a good use of it, unless you can fit storage boxes in the bottom. The Early Learning Centre has wardrobes with a lower rail that can be removed once the clothes become longer. Shelves will always be useful for toys, clothes, toiletries and books.

To maximize the space in a wardrobe, you can buy all-in-one Cubby Cubes — four colourful cubes, each holding up to 15lbs of clothes or accessories, available from the Great Little Trading Company catalogue twenty-four-hour order line on 0171 376

3337. They also have closet extenders, extra rails on a chain which hook on to the existing rail to double the storage space. The Bright Start catalogue (tel. 0171 483 3929), too, has useful items to help you make the best use of storage space.

The little hangers you can get free with women's underwear work well for baby clothes. Sometimes the hangers are offered to you when you buy baby clothes (always say yes). Otherwise Mothercare sells packs of children's hangers.

Toy Storage

Avoid toy chests unless they have:
- a special locking stay when opened;
- rounded edges;
- finger-trap gaps.

Even the light, wicker varieties have the potential to cause fatal accidents to toddlers. If you already have a toy chest, ensure that it is well ventilated and fix a stay from your local hardware store. Do It All sells stays for about £3.50.

Billie Bond Designs (mail order, tel. 01245 360164) make toy chests with the above safety features and Mothercare are planning to introduce them in 1996.

As well as being potentially dangerous, a toy chest guarantees chaos. The toy your toddler wants is always at the bottom, so the entire contents of the chest will probably be a permanent fixture on the nursery floor.

If you would rather have plastic storage boxes on wheels or castors, you can get the Easy Glide Store & Stock, a pack of two boxes and one set of castors, for £9.75. You can buy an extra set of castors for £1.69 and a lid for £1.99. These are available by mail order from Lakeland Plastics, tel. 015394 88100.

Imaginative, alternative storage ideas
- Make various-sized pigeonholes to store toys along one wall. This is educational for older children as it helps them

find the right-sized hole for a toy. These can be incorporated into a mural scheme as castle turrets, dolls' houses, etc.
- Suspend on very short strings coloured laundry bags beneath a shelf, each one labelled for a different use. The idea is that only one bag can be used at a time and has to be tidied away before the next one is used.

Controlling cuddly toys

If these seem to be breeding at an alarming rate, either of the following storage methods is appropriate until your baby is old enough and curious enough to try to reach them.
- A toy hammock – a white elasticated net hammock that can be hung from the wall or ceiling, price £6.99 from John Lewis or by mail order from First Choice (plus £2 postage and packing) on 01992 760911.
- A toy chain – a 72in chain with twenty fixed clothes pegs from which you can hang individual soft toys. It comes with a metal ceiling hook and screws, price £4.75 from Lakeland Plastics, tel. 01539 488100.

Children's Furniture

Stockists of child-sized furniture are as follows:

Debenhams' Junior Homestore Collection has two themes, toys and circuses. They have painted stools from £12.99 and tables from £39.99. Child-sized wicker chairs start at £19.99.

IKEA sell brightly coloured armchairs from £29; a pouffe table at £19. There are branches at Brent Park in north London, Croydon, Warrington, Gateshead and Birmingham. Tel. 0181 208 5600 for details.

Most good stores stock Little Tikes furniture in indestructible, safe, coloured plastic. There is a table and rocking-chair at £75.

The **Early Learning Centre** offer red plastic tables for £13.99 and matching chairs at £14.99 for two.

Freeman's catalogue sell a child's rocking-chair (£26.99).

Ring the order line on 0345 900 100. For a catalogue call 0800 900 200.

Contact **Dragons**, 23 Walton Street, London SW3, tel. 0171 589 3795, if you want what royal children have . . .

See also Chapter 4 on Safety.

13 Bedtime

Cots and Cotbeds

Cots

Before going shopping, measure the part of the room where you want the cot to go. Do not buy a model that is too big. If you are going to put the cot against a wall and you want one with a drawer underneath for storage, check that the drop-side device (the mechanism that enables you to lower one side of the cot) is on the same side as the drawer. Cots for under £50 which comply with the British Standard are available at Argos and Littlewoods. Most cots are sold without mattresses, so budget for this additional cost.

The medical establishment is divided as to how safe it is to sleep with your baby next to you in bed. Do not even consider it if you have had a few drinks or if you smoke in bed.

The Bed-Side-Bed from the Bed-Side-Bed Company, tel. 0181 989 8683, is a three-sided cot which fits against your bed (price £249.95). The fourth side is supplied for adding at a later date.

Never use a pillow for a baby under twelve months old.

Castors are useful for moving the cot to clean the floor.

Most cots have drop-side mechanisms, which allow you to lift the baby in and out easily. Some can be tricky to operate – try it out in the shop using one hand to check that you can fasten and unfasten it while holding the baby.

A two- or three-position base enables you to adjust the height of the mattress in the cot. Use the higher level when the baby is small so that you do not have to bend right down into the cot to reach her (a huge advantage for parents with back problems). The lower levels are for when your baby has grown sufficiently to climb or fall out.

A teething rail, a clear plastic edge which fits on to the sides of the cot, stops a teething baby from gnawing the woodwork.

What to look for

- The cot should comply with BS1753 1987.
- Something solid. A rickety cot is potentially lethal.
- Examine the base – even if it means spoiling the display in the shop. Take the mattress up and have a good look and feel. Is it really strong and secure? Will it cope with a baby bouncing up and down on it?
- Ask about assembly – you have to assemble many cots yourself. Can you cope with it or will it be too complicated for you?

Buying Second-Hand

- Be wary if you are buying the cot in dismantled form. Cots originally supplied in one piece can be damaged by being taken apart.
- Ensure that the original screws are supplied. The wrong type could cause the cot to collapse.
- Check the base for damaged springs or splits in the wood.
- Cracked or damaged side bars are hard to replace and could cause serious injury.
- Check that the bars, drop-side mechanism and supports on the base are in good condition.
- Don't use an old mattress. Invest in a new one. The gap between the mattress and the edge of the cot should be no bigger than 4cm (two fingers). Otherwise, there is a danger that the baby will get his head stuck.

- If you are going to repaint the cot, check that the paint is lead-free and non-toxic.
- Remove any decorative transfer on the inside to prevent choking if it peels off.
- There must be no bars or ledges that might help the baby climb out.

Cotbeds

A cotbed is a larger cot which converts into a bed when your baby is ready for one. The sides are taken off leaving the high bedhead and tailpiece. Some cots convert into other pieces of furniture, such as desks.

Do not buy one if you definitely do not intend to have another baby for at least two years, otherwise you will end up having to buy another cot for the second baby. On the other hand, if you plan to have another baby immediately, they are a good idea, as you will not have to kick a one-year-old out of her cot prematurely – you can simply change it into a bed when she is ready. Cotbeds are also often recommended as a sensible buy for twins and triplets, as each sibling can go at his or her own pace.

Do not buy a cotbed that is too babyish in design: an older child may find it offensive.

When your cot or cotbed is in use:
- Periodically check that all fastenings are secure and the cot is stable.
- Ensure that the drop-side mechanism is moving smoothly.
- When your baby is big enough to attempt to climb out, remove all large toys fixed on the cot sides so that she cannot use them as footholds.
- Make sure that your baby cannot reach any mobile.
- Never use a harness to secure your baby in the cot.
- Don't use bumpers with long ties or any toys with cords or ties longer than 20cm.

- Keep the assembly instructions in a safe place: you may have to put it away and bring it out again quite a few times.

Lead-free Paint for Cots

The Women's Environmental Network advice line (WENDI), tel. 0171 704 6800, suggests water-based paints rather than solvents. The following are natural and environmentally friendly paints:
- **Nutshell Natural Paints**, mail order from 01803 762329.
- **Auro**: telephone 01799 584888, or call the Woodmatters shop in north London on 0171 700 2638.
- **Biofa**: telephone 01865 374964.

Mattresses

If your cot does not come with its own mattress it should be labelled to tell you what size mattress to buy.

Safety update

There has been considerable concern about the link between cot mattresses and Sudden Infant Death Syndrome or cot death (see page 320). The government offers the following guidelines.

There is no single cause of cot death, but the best ways to protect your baby are:
- Do not let him get too hot – a room temperature of 18 degrees C (65 degrees F) and a covering of two cotton cellular blankets is fine. (You can buy nursery thermometers from Boots or Mothercare for £2.99.)
- Do not smoke during pregnancy or near your baby.
- Put him to sleep on his back.
- Do not use an old or second-hand mattress.
- If you are worried about your baby's health, contact your GP.

Buy your mattress from a reputable stockist such as Mothercare, John Lewis or a specialist retailer. New mattresses must meet BS1877 Part 10 1982. If there is any chance of your baby suffering from an allergy, your doctor will probably tell you that a fibre mattress is essential.

Unless you have an asthmatic baby, there is no particular ideal mattress. Mothercare advise that you buy the kind of mattress you would buy for yourself.

Some people believe that you must buy a mattress with vents otherwise air cannot circulate, which is dangerous. The truth of the matter is that air cannot circulate through the solid bottom of a cot anyway.

The two commandments for mattress buying are:
- It must fit your cot.
- It must be at least 10cm thick.

Foam Mattresses

These usually have holes at one end for ventilation and a PVC or mesh covering.

PLUS POINT
* Cheap.

MINUS POINT
* If the baby dribbles or vomits into the vents, the mattress can go mouldy, so you will need to clean it very thoroughly.

★★★ **Star buys** ★★★

Mothercare foam-interior mattresses start at £25.99.

Rochingham's Visivent Saferest, 10cm thick with a quilted cover, is available from £35.

Fibre Mattresses

PLUS POINTS
* Porous yet water-resistant. If a baby vomits or his nappy leaks, the fluid will drain away from him.
* Can go in the washing-machine and spin-drier.
* Hypoallergenic, so suitable for asthmatic babies.
* Contains no chemical fire-retardants.

MINUS POINT
* Some are expensive.

★★★ Star buy ★★★

Cotsafe Products mattresses – prices start from £35. Telephone 01625 501396 or write to Waters Green House, Waters Green, Macclesfield, Cheshire SK11 6LF.

Sprung Mattresses

These are foam mattresses containing springs for extra support.

PLUS POINT
* Hard-wearing.

MINUS POINT
* As with a foam mattress, you may have trouble cleaning these. Some come with fully removable quilted covers for cleaning (which cost around £9 extra).

★★★ Star buys ★★★

The Rochingham Kumfy Sprung with zip cover in quilted polypropylene, starts at £39.
   Early Learning Centre sprung mattresses from £32.99.
   Mothercare natural cotton with sprung interior, from £35.99.

Natural Coir/Coconut-Hair Mattresses

These are traditional, firm mattresses.

> **PLUS POINT**
> * Supportive.
>
> **MINUS POINT**
> * If you do not notice in time that your baby has soiled the mattress, liquid can penetrate to the core and necessitate a major cleaning exercise.

★★★ Star buy ★★★

Rochingham Golden Slumber coir wrapped in wool (from £50), which you can wash through with a shower attachment. The Early Learning Centre and Mothercare also do good-value versions.

If you are ordering a mattress over the telephone, you should know what the standard shapes are:

Square has right-angled corners.
Clipped has the corners 'clipped' off.
Round-cornered has the corners rounded of.
Oval has curved ends.

Mattress Covers

Some mattresses have a PVC side (e.g., some models from Mothercare, the Early Learning Centre, Relyon and Rochingham and Babywise) which you may want to use face up if your baby tends to posset. Alternatively you can buy a plastic mattress cover. Get a fitted one: the others can be dislodged and ruck up rather uncomfortably. Unfortunately, the waterproof-backed, towelling fitted sheet can take ages to dry as you cannot put it in the tumble-drier. Good brands are Playgro's Wetsafe waterproof cotton towelling protector (£9.99 for standard cot size – call 01536 523188 for stockists), or the Jonelle waterproof glove sheet (£7.50 from John Lewis).

Bedding

A combination of cotton cellular blankets and sheets is recommended by virtually all health professionals. You can add layers if the baby gets cold and take off layers if he is too hot. Do not be tempted to let him sleep under one of the pretty duvets displayed in the baby stores. Because they cannot be tucked in, they could ride up over his head.

You can save money by cutting down your own old sheets for the baby. Otherwise, you need:
- four cotton cellular blankets;
- four top sheets;
- four bottom or fitted sheets (terry, normal or brushed cotton).

Use a room thermometer to make sure the temperature in the baby's room is just right, and use the following guide to adjust his bedding.

27°C/80°F	Sheet only
24°C/75°F	Sheet and one layer of blankets*
21°C/70°F	Sheet and two layers of blankets
18°C/65°F	Sheet and three layers of blankets
15°C/60°F	Sheet and four layers of blankets
	*A double blanket counts as two layers

Cot Bumpers

Cot bumpers are padded strips that are tied on to the inside of a cot, shielding the baby's head from the cot bars. They are disliked by the Foundation for the Study of Infant Deaths (FSID) because they believe there is a danger of a tiny baby pressing his head against a bumper, which could lead to overheating, and of an older baby trying to use it to get out of the cot. The bumper ties are also perceived as a potential risk, though manufacturers are careful to keep them as short as possible.

Lambskin Fleeces

FSID have concerns about sheepskin as it is such a good insulator that it carries a risk of overheating the baby. However, no specific research has been done on this subject. Sheepskin fleeces are occasionally recommended for babies with skin problems.

Covered Foam Wedges

These keep a baby lying on his side. Avoid them as they can restrict natural movement. In any case, most medical professionals now advise that a baby should be laid down to sleep on his back.

Moses Baskets

Most Moses baskets are sold 'dressed', i.e., covered in fabric and with a quilt included in the price. The FSID recommends that you do not use the quilt: use cotton cellular blankets and a sheet instead.

Only buy a Moses basket if:
- You do not have a carrycot or baby carrier, i.e., you have no portable day bed for your baby and do not want to wheel your pram into the bedroom or kitchen.

- You find your carrycot or baby carrier too heavy to move around your home.
- You want a decorative bed to show off your new baby.
- You tend to take the carrycot out in all weathers so it is often damp when you come in and you do not yet have a cot for your baby.
- You are expecting more than one baby. If you are having to move more than one baby from room to room, Moses baskets are far lighter than carrycots.

If you do buy one, remember:

- Most babies grow out of their Moses baskets in a matter of weeks.
- They are not waterproof, so be wary of taking it outside.
- They are not a substitute for a pram and are unsuitable for use in a car.
- It is a complete waste of money to buy sheets to fit a Moses basket. Buy sheets to fit your cot and fold them as appropriate for the Moses basket.
- If you are going to leave your Moses basket on the floor, be sure that it is not in the path of draughts, pets or toddlers.

Moses baskets come in either wicker or palm. Wicker is more hard-wearing, so is often used for the larger baskets, but it tends to be more expensive. Palm is flexible and more reasonably priced. Check the hood carefully in the shop: some are very fiddly; others are not made with enough fabric, so you get a nasty gap at the back.

The bigger models are the best value as you can use them for a longer period of time.

Handles sewn down into the sides are stronger than those mounted on the top edge.

Clair de Lune make a wide selection from around £39.99, available from independent retailers. They are reasonably solid, good value and have a hood that works properly.

Stands

If you want to buy a wooden stand for your Moses basket and you cannot find a suitable one near you, ask your local independent baby shop to contact Saplings of Shropshire on 01630 639507.

Comforters and Soothers

Your baby may soothe himself by sucking a dummy, or a particular blanket or toy. Sixty per cent of children under the age of five are thought to use some sort of comforter.

If your baby is 'sucky' and does not have a comforter he might start sucking his thumb. The problem with this is that you cannot take it away.

Dental surgeon Susan Tanner, who has a large paediatric practice, says that there are two aspects of comforter use that concern dentists. First is the length of time a soother is in the baby's mouth; second, how vigorously the baby sucks. A soother in constant use by a vigorous sucker can cause teeth to stick out if the habit persists. If it is stopped before the child reaches four or five the teeth tend to revert to a neutral position. Any comforter that is used occasionally and is not sucked too strongly will cause minimal damage, if any.

If you do use a soother:

- Rinse and sterilize dummies as you would a bottle teat. The thrush virus, *candida albicans*, can get inside any small tear on the dummy and recurrently infect your baby's mouth.
- Never coat it in anything sweet, as this could lead to tooth decay.
- If it falls on the ground sterilize it before giving it back to your child.
- Do not lick it clean yourself.

- Try to have a few duplicates.
- Check it regularly for signs of tearing as this could present a choking hazard.
- If your baby uses a blanket as a comforter, throw it away if it gets ragged, as this too could cause choking.

PLUS POINTS
* Comforters are a stress-free way of settling your baby.
* Your child can soothe himself.
* You can control how much your baby uses it and when to get rid of it.

MINUS POINTS
* It is all too easy to start popping a soother in your baby's mouth whenever he is unhappy without establishing the reason for his misery.
* Some behavioural experts are concerned that dependence on a comforter over a long period will make a child slow to talk, socially awkward and fearful of exploring new textures with his mouth.

If you are going to buy a soother look for:
- An orthodontic teat – these disturb the shape of the mouth the least.
- Large holes in the plastic surrounding the teat so that saliva can drain away from the face. If it is trapped against the skin it can cause blisters.
- The British Safety standard 5239 1988, which guarantees that the dummy will be robust and non-toxic.

★★★ Star buy ★★★

If you buy the Avent hard blister pack of two (price £2.39), keep the box for when you have lost or destroyed the contents so that you can use it for storing cheaper soothers.

Baby Monitors

> *'I thought our new house was haunted until I realized that the lullabies and giggles I frequently heard were interference from another household on our baby monitor.'*
> **West London mother**

If you can hear your baby's cries from your sitting room, kitchen and bedroom, you do not need a monitor: they are for people who are out of earshot. If you plan to have your new baby with you during the day and sleeping in your room at night, wait a while and watch your friends' monitors in action to see whether you really need one. They are not foolproof. In the past, monitors were notoriously unreliable and retailers resigned themselves to the fact that they would receive a large number of returns. Newer models are better, but the success of the monitor depends very much on the user. If you live close to other families with monitors, you will probably pick up interference, although some models have a choice of two channels to minimize this. If babysitters and other members of the family will need to use the monitor, do not choose anything too complicated.

Some monitors come with integral night lights.

If you have a choice of channels, always check that both the baby's unit and your receiver are on the same one. If you get strange noises or interference, try the other channel. Place the unit out of the baby's reach but not more than 10ft (3m) from his cot. Units are not designed to be left outside in rain or extreme heat.

If you want a monitor that does not need batteries, look at plug-ins or rechargeables.

Plug-In Models

The baby unit is plugged into a standard socket within 10ft of baby. The listener's unit is connected to a socket in the room where you are. If you just need to listen out for the baby while you are watching TV in the living room or working in the kitchen, a plug-in will suit you fine.

Portables

The baby unit is either plugged in via an adaptor, or run off batteries. The listener's unit can also use either mains power or batteries. If you need to be able to wander around with the monitor, get a portable. You should be able to take the unit out into the garden or anywhere within 100m of the baby. Portables often come with a visual display. The Tomy Walkabout, for example, has an array of small lights which come on if your baby is crying. This is a useful feature if you do want to have the monitor on but do not want to be disturbed by your baby's every sound, for instance, if you are working from home.

If you need a monitor because you travel a lot and want to be able to leave it in, say, a hotel bedroom with your baby and listen in while you eat downstairs or sit outside, go into Tandy or a good consumer electrical shop and investigate walkie-talkies that cover more than 100m. Tandy produces a model with a range of one mile at £59.99 which works indoors and outside, and you have the choice of using batteries or the mains with an adaptor. Test any walkie-talkie for interference before you buy.

Rechargeables

These are basically the same as portables, except that they contain a sealed rechargeable battery which should last between two and three years. You can still use the monitor while the listener's unit is recharging.

Aerials
Aerials seem to hold an extreme fascination for toddlers, who seem to feel duty-bound to twang them every time they go past.

If you have an aerial that has been twanged to breaking-point, whether it is on a mobile phone or a monitor, Tandy and consumer electrical retailers sell a selection of bolt-on replacements, ranging in price from £9.99 to £24.99. Take your appliance into the shop to ensure that you buy the right one.

★★★ Star buys ★★★

The Tomy Walkabout 2000 (£29.99 at Mothercare and independent retailers) is a portable monitor with a visual display. It uses batteries but has a low-energy consumption, which is why we recommend this over the Tomy top-of-the-range monitor, the Recharge-About. This is £10 dearer but does not depend on batteries.

The Boots Chatterbaby plug-in (£21.99) is good value and works well. It also incorporates a nightlight.

Heartbeat monitors

Baby breathing monitors are used by FSID and the medical profession for babies who have breathing problems or by parents who need reassurance, for example those who have previously had a cot death. They are not recommended for healthy infants. Contact FSID if you have any queries about them.

PART SEVEN
EATING

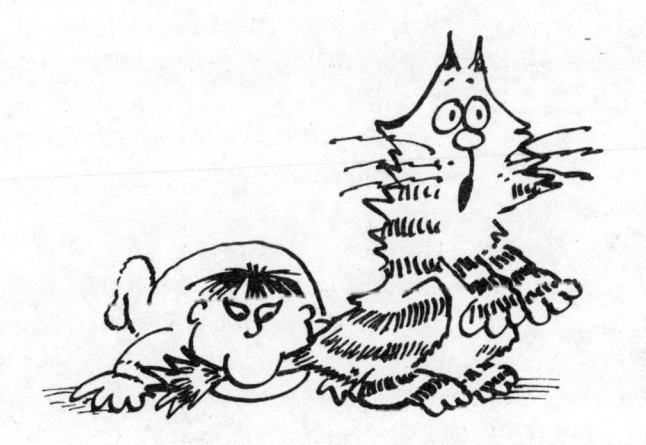

14   Feeding Your Baby

Breasts and Breastfeeding

Breastfeeding *is* bestfeeding. Breastmilk is the ultimate convenience food; it is also a complete and dynamic food, changing to meet your baby's needs. Above all, it is a uniquely protective food, for your baby and for you, his mother. Breastfeeding is about comfort and cuddles, about respecting and responding to your baby's needs, about believing in yourself and your body at an almost primitive level.

Getting it right can take practice, but your nipples and nerves can only stand so many near misses. There is no substitute for an expert – professional or lay – beside you to check your feeding position until you, and your baby, get the hang of it. If you're in hospital, ring the bell to ensure that a midwife watches you the first few times you put the baby to the breast.

If you keep forgetting which side you should start feeding with, attach a safety pin to the relevant bra strap and change it to the other side at the end of each feed to remind yourself.

At home, your community midwife will visit as often as necessary and should give you a contact number in case you need her help at other times. If you need extra guidance, at home or in hospital, an NCT or La Leche League breastfeeding counsellor is usually available to offer support by phone or in person. You do not have to be a member of either organization, but remember that both are charities and their counsellors are not paid, so donations to their head office are always welcome.

To find the name of your local breastfeeding counsellor call the head office of the NCT on 0181 992 8637, La Leche League on 0171 242 1278, or La Leche League of Ireland on 478 4885.

If you find breastfeeding difficult, remember you are not alone. Network; find out about coffee mornings and support groups and *go*. Build up a circle of other mothers whom you can call when the going gets tough. Having problems with breastfeeding does not mean you are any less a mother. Of course, your baby needs nourishment, but if, in the end, you cannot supply this yourself, it does not matter. He also needs love, security and fun – and it is much easier to offer these things when you yourself are happy and relaxed.

How to find out more

The NCT and La Leche League both offer a comprehensive range of leaflets on all aspects of breastfeeding. Telephone NCT Maternity Sales on 0141 633 5552 and write to La Leche League Books, 160 Blenheim Street, Hull HU5 3PN, for recent catalogues.

Further reading

Bestfeeding: Getting Breastfeeding Right For You by Mary Renfrew, Chloe Fisher and Suzanne Arms, Celestial Arts, Berkeley, California, £9.99. Excellent on positioning, with many helpful illustrations.

The NCT Book of Breastfeeding, Mary Smale, Vermilion, £8.99. A realistic, sympathetic look at all aspects of breastfeeding.

Successful Breastfeeding from the Royal College of Midwives, Churchill Livingstone, £5. Written for midwives and based firmly on modern research yet accessible to all.

Feeding in Public

...ding babies make ideal travelling and dining com-
...is perfectly possible to feed a small baby so discreetly

that people sitting just a few feet away will be unaware of it. Here's how:
- Wear a baggy top, preferably cool and made of cotton so that your baby can snuggle up underneath it. Avoid front-buttoned dresses and garments which involve pulling your breasts out through slits.
- Take a scarf or shawl to drape artistically over your shoulders and breasts – but watch out for little hands grabbing and pulling.
- If possible, choose your seat carefully; in a corner, by a window, beside a pot plant or close to other mothers are good positions.
- Take a friend for moral support.

Mentally rehearse what you would say if somebody should object. For example, 'My baby is very hungry. I think his crying would disturb people a lot more than his feeding.'

Friendly restaurants for breastfeeding mothers

A free booklet listing these is available from the Royal College of Midwives, 15 Mansfield Street, London W1M 0BE. Enclose an SAE.

Clothes for Breastfeeding

Don't bother with gimmicky nightwear with slits – you do not need any special maternity nightwear, just something that allows you to easily expose your breast, otherwise you will drip milk down your nightdress. Remember that the hospital will be hot, so buy breathable fabrics.

For the *dernier cri* in maternity nightwear, NCT mail-order sales (0141 633 5552) have nightshirts that co-ordinate with babywear. Grown-up nightshirts for men and women start at £17 and baby rompers at £4.75. Otherwise, high-street stores such as Mothercare, Marks & Spencer and John Lewis will have something suitable.

Avoid over-fussy nightwear – scratchy lace could irritate your baby's skin. Suitable 'gowns' are available by mail order from Mele of London, tel. 0171 732 7263.

Rugby shirts with 'invisible' zips for breastfeeding are obtainable from Blooming Marvellous mail order.

Breast Pads

For some women, the sound of a baby crying – any baby – is enough to bring milk gushing forth in spectacular fashion. If you do tend to leak:
- Use breast pads inside your bra.
- Wear dark or patterned tops.
- Sleep on a towel at night.
- In an emergency, fold up a thin sanitary towel or a large cotton handkerchief and slip it inside your bra.

Breast pads come in many forms: round, square, shaped, flat, disposable, washable, white, beige. It is impossible to recommend the ultimate breast pad because mothers' breasts and needs vary so much. Be warned: these small pads do seem to have a life of their own and you can find them wandering out of your sleeves at the most inappropriate moments.

Disposables

The two brands which come in for consistent praise from consumers are Johnson's nursing pads (£3.49 for fifty) and Boots' shaped breast pads (£2.89 for fifty). Both are circular and contoured and seem to stay in place. Johnson & Johnson's were preferred by women with light leakage; they have no plastic layer and therefore allow the skin some breathability.

Reusables

If you are ecologically friendly – or, indeed, financially challenged – reusable breast pads are worth trying. The most absorbent seem to be Emma Jane non-disposables. Ameda reusable nursing pads (£6 for six) are also good; Boots' and Mothercare's washable pads are cheaper at around £4 for a half-dozen.

Breast Shells

These are semi-spherical, plastic devices of limited use. If milk spurts out of one breast while you are feeding from the other you may wish to collect it in a breast shell. You could chill or freeze this milk for use later, but remember that it is only relatively low-calorie foremilk. If you plan to collect milk in this way, breast shells must be carefully cleaned and sterilized. A pair of shells costs around £4.

Nipple Shields

These small, flexible plastic items, strongly reminiscent of sombrero hats, are designed to fit over your nipple and part of the surrounding areola during feeding. They may be useful if you have very sore or cracked nipples, since they form a barrier between your nipple and the baby. However, nipple shields should be used with extreme caution: they easily distract from correct positioning of the baby at the breast and it can be very difficult to wean your baby from them later. They cost around £3 a pair.

Nipple Cream

Your nipples and areolae come fully equipped with their own built-in moisturizers. Generally, man-made creams, lotions and sprays are superfluous, and some may be a potential source of skin irritations and allergic reactions. Furthermore, research has shown that babies recognize their mother's milk and breast by smell and therefore favour unwashed and unanointed breasts. Sore nipples are best dealt with by paying careful attention to the position of the baby's mouth on your breast and by rubbing a little of your milk (which has amazing antiseptic and healing properties) on to your nipples after each feed.

If you do feel a proprietary cream would be soothing, then go for Lansinoh, a 100 per cent natural, hypoallergenic cream that does not need to be removed before breastfeeding. Tel. Egnell Ameda on 01823 336362 for details. Prices from £3.50.

Cabbage leaves

Soothe engorgement with cool flannel compresses, or try placing cold cabbage leaves inside your bra. *Gently* express a little milk before feeding to soften the breast.

Milk Expression and Breast Pumps

> *'I stopped storing breastmilk in the fridge when I realized that the builders were using it in their coffee.'*
> **South London mother**

One of the many joys of breastfeeding is the delightful absence of clutter and equipment. However, many mothers do eventually find that they want the flexibility offered by expressing milk for somebody else to give to their baby later. This might be just once a month for a special evening out, or every day during the working week. Try to avoid bottles and teats (and dummies) for the first four to six weeks of breastfeeding. During this time you and your baby are still consolidating breastfeeding skills and the use of teats can cause considerable disruption, simply because the technique of bottle feeding is so different from that of breastfeeding. If you need to give breastmilk indirectly in the early weeks, consider using a dropper, spoon or small cup such as those produced by Ameda (£2.85 for three).

Many women find milk expression easy and effortlessly produce rows of brimming bottles for the babysitter. Others find the whole business difficult and embarrassing. You may find milk spurting from your breasts when your baby is wriggling on your lap, only to dry up completely when faced with an expensive collection of cold glass and plastic tubes. For this reason, probably the most effective way to express milk is to pump one breast while you are feeding your baby from the other, perhaps during an early-morning feed.

Manual Expression

This method is simplicity itself insofar as you need only clean hands and a sterile wide-necked bowl. It is surprisingly effective apparently once you have the knack, but considerable time and practice is needed to achieve good results. Ask your midwife or health visitor for details or send for La Leche League's explanatory leaflet. Even if you have a pump, it is a useful technique to know for emergencies.

Pumps

Breast pumps are sold in most babycare shops and chemists. Look for the usual high-street brands, plus Avent, Pur Natur and Pigeon. The Ameda range is available by mail order, either through the NCT or direct from Egnell Ameda, tel. 01823 336362.

If you buy a pump ask the shop or supplier whether they will refund your money if you cannot make it work for you.

If you want to be absolutely certain that expressing will work, and money is no object, it is worth hiring a large powered pump. These work for most people. But do not dismiss the more cost-effective options out of hand.

Hand pumps

These may have a lever or a syringe action, with the milk being collected in either an attached bottle or in the cylinder of the pump itself. Hand pumps are cheap, quiet, portable and relatively discreet, but most need two – strong – hands to operate them. They cost between £9 and £18, and are good for occasional use.

Small powered pumps

These are usually battery operated, though some have a mains lead. They can be rather noisy to use, but still quite compact and portable. Look for pumps with a range of settings and an automatic 'surge' action which mimics the baby's suckling. Powered pumps are rather more expensive at £30 to £50, excluding (lots of) batteries.

Large powered pumps

The large versions are mains-operated, efficient and comparatively quiet, but very expensive (£500 to £700), and about as discreet and as portable as an electric sewing machine. You can hire one from local breastfeeding organizations for about £1 a day plus around £8.50 to buy your own collection kit.

Storing Expressed Milk

Expressed breastmilk must be handled with care. All containers and pump components which come in contact with it should be scrupulously cleaned and sterilized. If you are using bottles and other equipment only occasionally do not waste money on a sterilizer: instead put cleaned bottles and teats in a pan of boiling water. Make sure that they are totally immersed and filled with water and boil for ten minutes.

Expressed milk should be chilled immediately in a fridge or good coolbox or bag and used within two days. Breastmilk can also be frozen, but remember that freezing destroys its unique antibodies. Fresh milk is vastly superior.

The choices for chilling and freezing breastmilk include:
- Wide-necked breast milk-storage bottles, such as Boots'

model. These have squared-off edges to fit neatly into the fridge (£5.49 for four).
- A sterilized ice-cube tray is especially good for freezing small amounts for a young baby.
- Pre-sterilized freezer bags (£7 for twenty at Boots) can be defrosted later and the contents emptied into a feeding bottle.
- Pre-sterilized freezer bags (£3.99 for twenty) which fit straight into a bottle system, such as Avent's.

Look out for specially designed breast-pump coolbags for carrying around your pump, expressed milk and other bits and pieces. Both Ameda and Boots sell them, at £14.50 and £12.99 respectively.

For excellent advice and service on all things to do with breastfeeding, call Felicity Tucker at Mothernature, on 0161 485 7359. Felicity is a trained breastfeeding counsellor and she can supply bras and pumps.

Further reading

Send for *A Mother's Guide to Milk Expression and Breast Pumps*, *Manual Expression of Breast Milk: Marmet Technique* and *Breastfeeding your Baby: A Guide for Working Mothers*, all three from La Leche League, and *How to Express and Store Breast Milk* from the NCT. All are leaflets costing between 60p and £1.

This section was written with assistance from Hannah Hulme Hunter SRN RM, midwife and mother.

Bottle Feeding

Breastfeeding may be the optimum method of feeding a new baby, but for some mothers, it just is not possible. Don't let other people make you feel guilty about it. If your baby is obviously not thriving on breastmilk, consult your community midwife or health visitor: formula milk may prove to be as soothing to your nerves as it is to his stomach.

The secret of relaxed bottle feeding is to have a routine. Sterilize bottles and prepare feeds for the next twenty-four hours at a set time daily. Most people find this easiest to do just before they go to bed at night or first thing in the morning, putting the bottles in the sterilizer before breakfast and making up the feeds immediately afterwards. Once you have allowed the contents to cool, the bottles *must* stay in the fridge. Warm them up as you need them, instead of frantically preparing bottles at odd hours of the day and night. Never keep formula in the fridge for longer than twenty-four hours, and if your baby does not finish a feed throw the remainder away as it will have been contaminated by his saliva.

Formula Milks

If you are bottle feeding in hospital and your baby seems content, stick with the same brand. The most popular makes in Britain are Boots' own brand, Cow & Gate, Farley's, Milupa and SMA.

There are three 'stages' of milk. Stage 1 has a whey base. If, after a couple of months, a baby does not seem satisfied by this, try stage 2, which is based on a protein called casein which takes longer to digest, and therefore makes the baby feel fuller. As many health professionals disapprove of giving cow's milk to babies under a year old, follow-on milks (stage 3) have been developed for babies who are on solid food. However, there is no nutritional reason to change to stage 3 from stage 2.

If formula milks seem to be giving your baby stomach upsets or causing allergies of any kind, you may be prescribed a soya-based milk. This is available on the NHS.

Popular Formula Milks

Make	Type		Cost
Boots	Stage 1:	Formula 1	£5.09 900g
	Stage 2:	Formula 2	£5.09 900g
	Stage 3:	Follow-on Milk	£5.09 900g
Cow & Gate	Stage 1:	Premium	£5.69 900g
	Stage 2:	Plus	£5.69 900g
	Stage 3:	Step-up	£5.69 900g
Farley's	Stage 1:	First Milk	£4.93 900g
	Stage 2:	Second Milk	£4.93 900g
	Stage 3:	Follow-on Milk	£4.93 900g
Milupa	Stage 1:	Aptamil with Milupan	£5.99 900g
	Stage 2:	Milumil	£5.99 900g
	Stage 3:	Forward	£5.99 900g
SMA	Stage 1:	Gold	£5.75 900g
	Stage 2:	White	£5.75 900g
	Stage 3:	Progress	£5.75 900g
Soya milk	Wysoy (made by SMA)		£8.49 860g
	Intasoy (Cow & Gate)		£7.35 900g

Bottles

Feeding bottles are fast becoming designer items. Your child can suck on a giraffe, teddy or elongated Polo mint, but these glamour models are not ideal for infants, or for those attempting to feed them.

For infants buy standard bottles, narrow bottles that hold up to 250ml (9oz). Wide-necked bottles hold the same amount of milk but are stubbier and wider. They may leak from the lid when carried around, and can prove too chunky for older babies who want to feed themselves.

You can buy 4oz sizes in both the above designs, but you do not need these unless you intend to give your baby cooled, boiled water between feeds. However, you might want to buy this smaller version if you are expressing breast milk: you might feel much more positive about it if you can fill a bottle.

For older babies there are grip bottles with handles they can hold, but a baby should be using a trainer cup anyway by the time she is one year old. Drinking systems, versatile bottles that come with a teat and spout to convert from a bottle into a trainer cup, are expensive.

You can manage with four 9oz bottles but six is a good idea. Always have two extra teats around as old ones tend to split. A bottle brush is essential to thoroughly clean your bottles before you sterilize them.

Look for bottles which are:
- Easy to clean. Wider bottles are easier to clean and to fill, and breast-fed babies tend to adapt to wider teats more readily.
- Unlikely to leak. Some bottles can only be shaken when the teat is pointing down into the milk and a special sealing disc is screwed on the top like a lid. Look for the word 'self-sealing'.
- Good value. Don't waste money on a fancy design which may prove difficult to clean.
- Sterilizer-friendly. Not all bottles fit into all sterilizers, though standard bottles should be fine.

★★★ Star buy ★★★

Mothers, health visitors and nannies to whom we spoke were mainly in favour of the Avent brand. They found these bottles by far the easiest to hold and clean. They are by no means the cheapest, but may well be worth the extra expense – after all, getting milk into your baby is essential to her survival.

Boots, Mothercare and Tommee Tippee all produce good-value bottles and you can always try out a more expensive teat, such as the Nuk, on the standard-shaped versions of these.

Teats

Ignore all teat hype. There are wide-necked teats, orthodontic teats, pump-action teats and doubtless many others. As you cannot interview babies, there is no way of really knowing whether the manufacturers' claims for these wonders are true or otherwise. Just observe the following rules:

- The teats must fit your bottles. Check this before you buy.
- Where there is a choice of slow, medium or fast flow, start with the slow flow – you can always move up a stage. Milk coming through too fast can cause your baby to choke.
- Silicone teats are better value and last longer than the softer latex ones, though your baby may dislike them.
- If you go for latex, ensure that your baby does not nibble holes in it.

★★★ Star buy ★★★

Maws Resolve teats for standard bottles only are suitable for all flow speeds. These have a cross cut to allow the baby to control the flow rate and prevent colic. They are available at Boots for £1.90 for three.

NUK and Mothercare also produce orthodontic teats which may be more appealing to breastfed babies. If these are not accepted, or the baby cannot feed without dribbling much of her milk out of her mouth, try the Pur Natureflow teat (£1.99 for two for wide-necked bottles or £1.79 for two standard).

Disposable Systems

These are pre-sterilized bags which attach to a holder. All you have to do is to fill the bag with milk and push on a disposable teat. Disposable systems work out very expensive, but might be worthwhile for travellers who do not have access to a sterilizer. There are three manufacturers: Playtex, Pur and Avent. The Playtex system is extremely popular in the United States, where it is thought that there is less of a risk of colic when the baby is fed out of a bag rather than a bottle.

The Playtex starter kit (£6.50) consists of three holders, three rings, three caps and roll of fifty liners. Extra liners are £2.50 for fifty.

The Pur disposable feeding system provides two bottle-holders and forty liners for £8.99.

If you already have Avent bottles, the Avent disposable feeding bottle (bottle-holder, ten bags, one teat) at £3.99 is good for travelling. The teats are interchangeable, so your baby will not know the difference.

Boots sell a pack of ten disposable teats (£3.99) which fit straight on to their bottled drinks.

Bottle-Warmers

You can take the chill off your baby's milk by standing the bottle in a jug of hot water or by turning it gently under a hot tap. However, if the idea of doing this at 4 a.m. appals you, you may be tempted to buy a bottle-warmer. Some are designed to warm bottles only, others will warm baby food as well.

Do not rely on the bottle-warmer to heat the milk to the correct temperature — some heat the milk more vigorously than others. Shake the bottle to even out the temperature, and test it by placing a few drops on the back of your hand. It should be the same temperature as your skin.

You should not heat up bottles or food in a microwave oven. Although a bottle may feel cool when you take it out of the oven, the milk continues to heat up and can therefore become far too hot. Some babies have had their mouths badly scalded in this way.

If you have to use the microwave:
- Always leave the bottle to stand for at least two minutes after removing it from the oven.
- Shake the bottle well after heating.
- Test the temperature of the milk before feeding it to your baby.

> **!!!** Do not in any circumstances:
> * Keep milk warm for more than twenty minutes before a feed. If the baby does not want it, throw it away.
> * Put a warm bottle into an insulated bottle-holder or vacuum flask. Put a cold bottle into the flask and warm it when you need it.
> * Allow your travel bag to stay unwashed if milk has leaked into it. Old milk is a source of bacteria.

★★★ Star buys ★★★

The Avent bottle- and babyfood-warmer (£19.95) is safe and efficient.

The Boots bottle- and baby food-warmer (£17.99) is similar and cheaper.

The Babytec Electronic bottle- and food-heater (£18.95) cuts heating times by half but does not have a bowl option for baby food.

The Playskool night-time feeder (£12.95) is excellent if you want to heat bottles only.

Travelling Warmers

The Babytec car bottle- and food-heater (£9.95) plugs into a car cigar lighter but takes fifteen to twenty minutes to heat up water. It is not particularly efficient with wide bottles.

The Childcare travel bottle-warmer (£14.99 from independent retailers) uses crystal energy, so no batteries or electricity are needed.

Bolt-On Extras

It you want to attach a bottle to a pushchair, you can buy Attach-a-Bottle from Tomy (£1.99). This has a bottle-sized ring at one end with a press-stud fastening at the other to attach to a buggy or highchair. BabyBud manufactures Bottlebud, a clamp and ring which will securely hold the bottle on most baby carriers, buggies and prams. This comes in five colours to co-ordinate with your conveyance. Cosybud holds standard bottle flasks and Travelbud attaches to car doors. Bear in mind that such items may encourage snacking between mealtimes. You can buy BabyBud at Tesco. Call 01926 403131 for other stockists.

Sterilizers

The cheapest way to sterilize feeding equipment is to immerse it in boiling water in a large covered pan for at least ten minutes.

Chemical Sterilizers

This traditional sterilizer is a plastic tank which you fill with sterilizing fluid or water containing sterilizing tablets. You can use any airtight plastic container if you don't need to sterilize frequently.

PLUS POINTS
* Cheap initial outlay.
* Can be used anywhere – all you need is water.

MINUS POINTS
* It takes thirty minutes to sterilize bottles.
* Everything must be thoroughly rinsed in boiled water after sterilization to eliminate any residue.
* You need a supply of sterilizing solution or tablets. The cost of these works out at around £20 per year based on using the sterilizer twice a day for a year. If you are going to have more than one child, it is not cost-effective.
* The solution has to be changed every twenty-four hours.
* Some units are bulky.

Steam Sterilizers

You pour a measure of water into the unit, plug it in and steam is generated. This destroys bacteria. Try to find out through your local NCT if there are any second-hand models available. If you do buy one, check that it has the water-measuring cup with it. If not, establish the precise quantity of water required and measure it out using the scale on the side of a feeding bottle. If you live in a hard water area, descale your sterilizer regularly to keep both it and your bottles in mint condition.

PLUS POINTS
* It takes only about ten minutes.
* No special solutions are needed.
* Some units take up to six bottles, so you can prepare a day's feed.

MINUS POINTS
* The cost: most are over £30.
* They are large.
* They can mark bottles.

Microwave Sterilizers

These are based on the steam method, adapted for use with a microwave oven.

PLUS POINTS
* They take only ten minutes.
* The units are small and can be put away when not in use.
* No chemicals are involved.
* They are cheaper than steam sterilizers.

MINUS POINTS
* Some take only two or three bottles, which is a bore if every feed involves a bottle.
* They may be too big for your microwave. (Taking out the turntable can help.)
* You must wash the unit between uses.

Travelling

If you are travelling with a baby, you have a number of options to ensure that you are able to sterilize equipment properly.
- Take your own sterilizer with an adaptor if required.
- Use travel bags with tablets, available from John Lewis.
- Use a disposable bottle system.

Bibs

Even a baby who is only on milk can mess up his clothes in a dramatic fashion. Many people start off by simply wrapping a nappy muslin round the baby, but you will have to buy bibs sooner or later, so you might as well enjoy their benefits from an early stage. Any of the following provide maximum cover for a baby who is not yet on solids.

- **Terry-towel bibs.** The best ones for babies have velcro fastenings. They can be washed at high temperatures so removing all stains.
- **Plastic-backed bibs.** The plastic backing prevents dampness from seeping through to the baby's clothes. However, it also melts at high temperatures, so you cannot launder them in too hot a wash. If you are worried about permanent stains, choose heavily patterned items.
- **Plastic overalls.** Babies grow out of these quickly but they do provide full-scale protection.
- **Pelican bibs.** These rigid plastic bibs with shelves are most mothers' favourite. One wipe and they are clean. However, their stiff collars make them unsuitable for new babies.
- **Disposable bibs.** It is worth having one packet of these on hand for travelling or emergencies when all other bibs are in the wash.
- **Napkin clips.** These transform an ordinary paper or cloth napkin into a bib. Two fun clips on a ribbon (£4.50 each or £7.50 for a pack of two) can easily be kept in your bag. They are obtainable from Bright Start mail-order catalogue on 0171 483 3929.

Support While Feeding

Some people recommend V-shaped pillows, either to support your back or tucked across your waist to support the arm holding the baby. These are available at Argos (the Dunlop Bedtimer relaxer pillow is £4.79, pillowcase £3.29) and Littlewoods Index (Nightfall support pillow £4.99, pillowcase £3.50).

For information on dealing with colic, see Chapter 19.

Baby Foods

In many countries, the concept of special baby food does not exist. Babies eat what their families eat, mashed to a suitable consistency. Packaging foods in dear little bottles is just a marketing ploy that earns considerable sums for the manufacturers.

Dr Gillian Harris, clinical psychologist and lecturer at the University of Birmingham, recently completed a study into babies' food preferences which showed that even if a baby initially reacts with disgust to a food, he can learn to accept it provided that it is offered consistently.

'We found that mothers who gave their babies puréed family meals from an early age had fewer problems later on. So if you are keen for your baby to like nutritious foods such as avocado, do not be discouraged by a negative reaction. You should be able to gradually increase the quantity, starting with tiny amounts at first, until your baby acquires the taste.'

Dr Harris's guidelines for successful weaning

- Introduce a wide variety of foods as early as four months – babies enjoy different tastes. Our research shows that they can distinguish subtle alterations in flavours which adults cannot detect.
- If you are concerned about food allergies ask your health visitor for advice.

- If your baby does not appear to enjoy food, stay calm and take it slowly.
- Never put food in a baby's mouth when he is crying.
- Do not impose your own ideas of what is tasty and what isn't. We believe that mothers may be less likely to persevere with foods if they do not like them themselves.
- Do not leave it too late to introduce solids. Babies weaned after four months are likely to be lighter and to accept a smaller range of foods.

When you start introducing solids into your baby's diet you do not have to sterilize all feeding equipment, but make sure that all items are thoroughly washed, preferably in the washing-machine, where the water temperature is high enough to kill off most bacteria. Use kitchen paper or a clean dishcloth to dry feeding paraphernalia.

Be particularly vigilant about sell-by dates on baby foods and check that the seals are intact on baby-food jars. If you know that your baby will only eat half a jar of food, do not leave the unwanted half hanging around outside the fridge. Cover it up and put it inside immediately.

Home-Made Baby Food

You should phase in foods one at a time, so that you can be sure that your baby is not allergic to any particular substances, and identify it if he is. This is more likely if other members of your immediate family have a particular food allergy. Symptoms are vomiting, diarrhoea, colic, asthma and eczema. The most common allergies are to:
- egg whites;
- cow's milk;
- wheat cereals – look for gluten-free labels on processed baby foods.

Do not introduce any of these until your baby is six months old.

Equipment

You will need a sieve and a wooden spoon. If you are going to make food in large quantities for the freezer, you will need a food processor, freezer bags and ice-cube trays.

★★★ Star buy ★★★

Kenwood hand blender (Argos catalogue, £14.50). You can use this in the saucepan to blend tiny quantities of left-overs from your own meal.

Suitable fruits and vegetables are: apples, pears, peaches, bananas, dried fruit, broccoli, butternut squash, carrots, cauliflower, courgettes, green beans, swede, turnip, parsnip, peas and spinach.

Cut up fruit and vegetables into small pieces, removing skin, pips and blemishes, and steam, microwave or simmer in a little water until soft. Dried fruit will take the longest. Be careful not to overcook fruit and vegetables, or use too much water, or you may destroy the nutrients in the food. Rub it through a sieve or blend until smooth.

Consider adding a little breast milk or formula to give a creamy texture. Add baby rice with the milk to improve the texture of water purées.

Fruits which can be eaten raw are bananas, mashed to a creamy consistency with breast milk or formula; avocado; kiwi fruit which has been well sieved to exclude black seeds and core; soft pears and peaches.

Unsuitable foods

Remember that healthy-eating guidelines aimed at adults are not applicable to infants. Fats, for example, are an important energy-giving part of a baby's diet.

Too much fibre can reduce your baby's ability to absorb the other nutrients and calories he needs.

Avoid spicy, sugary, salty or smoked foods. These can put a strain on your baby's kidneys and digestive system.

When you have cooked and puréed the food, allow it to cool. Put it in an ice-cube tray inside a freezer bag in the freezer. One cube should be more than enough for each first meal. To serve, defrost the cube at room temperature, or overnight in the fridge if the food is intended to be served in the morning. Heat it until it is cooked through and then allow it to cool down before giving it to the baby.

Manufactured Baby Food

Feeding your baby from jars or tins is the infant equivalent of fast food. Ignore labels which claim, 'suitable for babies from 3–4 months' – not all babies have started on solids at four months.

The general rule is: the fewer the ingredients, the purer the baby food.

The Food Commission is unhappy about the use on food labels of terms like 'wholesome', 'nutritious', and 'natural goodness'. They feel that these words could persuade parents that foods prepared at home are not as well balanced as the bought varieties.

Do not buy first-stage foods that contain sugars (dextrose and fructose are added sugars), gluten or additional fillers such as starches or maltodextrin.

Do not assume that you are necessarily buying the picture on the jar. Look at the list of ingredients first. They are always listed in order according to how big a percentage of the contents they represent. The first item given is the main ingredient, the last is the smallest.

★★★ Star buys ★★★

The Baby Organix range, stocked by Sainsbury, ASDA, Safeway, Waitrose, CRS, William Low and health-food shops, avoids additives.

Boots Mother's Recipe (do not confuse this with their other range, First Harvest).

Heinz Pure Fruit is a variety of puréed fruits without additives available in tins and jars. HiPP, available at Boots and Tesco. Beechnut, an exceptional range from the USA, is only sold by a few outlets but if you can find it, it is well worth trying.

Cow's milk

Take advice from your health visitor on how cow's milk should be introduced into your baby's diet. At present, most dieticians recommend that only limited quantities should be used until your baby is over one year old and that only breast or formula milk should be used throughout his first twelve months. However, ideas on this subject change frequently. Goat's or sheep's milk, available at your supermarket, can be used as an alternative.

Feeding

The best way to introduce solids is to start with a teaspoon of non-wheat cereal, such as Milupa pure baby rice (£1.65 for 150g), mixed with breast or formula milk. Remember that it may take a while for your baby to get used to a spoon.

Cow & Gate produce an excellent wallchart on weaning, the Babyfeeding Guide, which is part of their In Touch programme. Ask for pack 3, Feeding – The First Six Months. Telephone 01225 768381 for further details, or write to Cow & Gate In Touch programme, FREEPOST 492, Trowbridge, Wiltshire B14 0YY, stating when your baby is due and whether this is your first pregnancy.

Equipment

You need a feeding spoon and a bowl – the lid of a feeding bottle is the perfect size, or use an egg cup.

★★★ Star buys ★★★

The Maws weaning spoon (£2.99 for three) changes colour to show if food is too hot. Testers found that it took a while to return back to its normal colour.

The Maws weaning food storage jars (£1.99 for a twin pack of two 4oz jars) are freezer-, microwave- and dishwasher-safe.

Highchairs and Baby Diners

When you first start weaning your baby on to solids, you will probably want to hold her on your lap or feed her in her bouncy chair or car seat. A baby should be able to sit up properly before you put her in a chair.

Highchairs

Some people suggest waiting until your baby is six months old before buying a highchair so that you can test the chair with her in it. But the person it has to suit is you.

What to look for

- Can you clean it easily?
- Will it take up too much room?
- Is it easy to assemble and store?
- Is it good value?
- Does it have D-rings so that you can attach a five-point harness if one is not incorporated? This is essential.
- Is it stable?
- Will your baby's plates and bowls fit on the tray?
- Does it have a good-size lip to stop plates falling off?

- Can the tray be adjusted or removed?
- Can you alter its height so that it can be drawn up to the table when the baby is older?

The best-value highchairs to be found include the Casdon Wooden highchair with white tray, at £23.99 from independent retailers and the Argos catalogue, and the Mothercare ABC Travel highchair, a real bargain at £29.99. It is strong, lightweight and can be folded flat for easy storage.

Country-Cottage-Style Highchairs

These are attractive, old-fashioned highchairs made of wood. They are sturdy, easy to clean and will last for years, but they do not fold away. You may want to buy a padded insert (£14.99 at Children's World) so that your baby is not uncomfortable on the hard seat. Generally speaking, the lip on the food trays is not as deep as on other types of highchair.

If you can still find a Continenta Cottage or Country Highchair at your local retailer, these are very attractive. They cost £84.95. The Mothercare Country Style highchair (£79.99) has the benefit of converting easily into an older child's table and chair. The Silver Cross Chatsworth (£79.99) is available at Children's World and independent retailers.

Multi-Position Highchairs

These have a number of adjustable height positions which allow them to be used by both babies and small children. The chair can also be used without its tray at the table, making it ideal for older children up to the age of ten or twelve.

★★★ Star buys ★★★

Mamas & Papas Futura, price £75.

Cosco, £27.75 from the Argos catalogue, is excellent value.

Folding Highchairs

These usually fold flat so that you can lean them against a wall when they are not in use. Some can be folded and collapsed to go into the car.

★★★ **Star buys** ★★★

The EastCoast folding highchair, which costs £57 from Children's World and independent retailers.

The Pine Foldaway, at around £50 from the Early Learning Centre and Mothercare.

For travelling in the car, the Mothercare Bambino (£39.99) folds to a compact size and the Britax Picnic (£49.50) folds into its own carrying bag.

High/Low Chairs

These convert from a conventional highchair to a low child's chair and table. They can be bulky but are adored by some children.

★★★ **Star buys** ★★★

Early Learning Centre convertible, £59. Cube highchair from the Argos catalogue, £37.99, is good value.

Highchair/Booster Seat

A highchair/booster seat (£29.99), with detachable tray that folds flat for travel and can be washed in the dishwasher, is available from the Great Little Trading Company mail order, tel. 0171 376 3337.

Baby Diners

There are several styles of baby seats that fix on to a dining table. A good sturdy design has a fabric or synthetic bucket-style seat on a metal frame which screws on to the table. Those lacking a proper screw mechanism are more prone to collapse. These chairs will not fit on to tables with a lipped edge.

The Royal Society for the Prevention of Accidents does not like baby diners because the safety of the chair depends on the stability of the table. So if you do get one ensure that:
- Your table is extremely stable and solid.
- Your baby wears a five-point harness in the seat.
- You check that the seat is secure every time you use it.

The advantages are:
- Your baby is sitting at the table with you, so you do not have to keep swivelling round to feed her.
- She is part of the family mealtime, which can be fun for everyone.
- If you do not have much space, you do not have to bother putting them away as they do not take up any room.
- They are very useful for travelling.

★★★ Star buy ★★★

Tommee Tippee Tota chair, available from independent retailers and John Lewis stores, price £27.75.

Other Options

Harnesses

Fabric harnesses with velcro straps for use with a normal chair can be called upon when there is no highchair around, but these are not advisable until the baby can support herself, at around six months. Sit'n'Secure, from the Bright Start catalogue, tel. 0171 483 3929, costs £12.95.

The Mothercare System 5 Supersitter

A multi-purpose option that is well worth considering, this is in turn a baby gym, swing, rocker, recliner and low chair, and last but not least, a highchair. It costs £99.99. If you can't get to a Mothercare, you will find it in their First Baby Guide and you can order it by telephone on 01923 240365.

'Splat' Mats

If you want to protect your floors and carpets, look out for PVC highchair floor mats, which start at around £6. Splat mats often come as free gifts with baby magazines.

PART EIGHT
GETTING AROUND

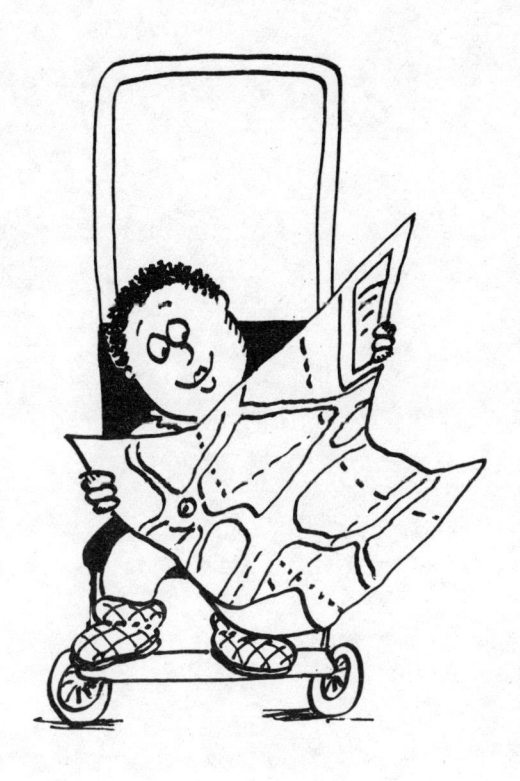

15 Baby Transport

Slings

A sling is a practical way of carrying a baby around, both in and out of doors, as it enables him to feel close to you without restricting your arms. You have three options: a baby-carrier that can be worn on either the chest or the back; a carrier that can adapt to a number of positions; or a backpack, for a baby old enough to support himself. Slings are useful if you often use public transport, go on frequent country walks or visit busy markets with poor access for prams; if you need to wheel an older child in a buggy while you carry your newborn, or if your partner wants to use it to bond with the baby.

It is much better to wait until the baby arrives before buying a sling, as only then can you be sure that it offers both the carrier and the carried the support they need. It can be a very expensive piece of kit, so you need to be sure you will use it. To hire one for a week costs around £7.

If your baby is a dribbler, look for a carrier with a detachable bib or one that is machine-washable. A headrest will stop the baby leaning back and upsetting your balance – most accidents with slings and backpacks happen when adults fall over.

You may be more comfortable with a sling that supports the baby on your hip.

What to look for
- Security. Some slings make you feel as if you need to hold on to your baby's head. You need to feel totally confident

that your baby's body is held securely to your own.
- Does it support the baby's lower half sufficiently?
- Well-padded shoulder straps and a waist belt make the carrier more comfortable.
- Does it suit the climate? Some have weatherproof covers.
- Is it comfortable for all adults who will be using it? If both you and your partner are going to use it, you should both go to the store to choose it.
- How easy is it to take on and off when there is no one to help? If you are buying a backpack, a carrier that can stand unsupported is generally the best buy.
- If you intend to use it a lot, choose one with a heavy fabric to minimize wear and tear.

★★★ Star buys ★★★

The Baby Bjorn, £39.95 at Boots.

If you don't like clips and buckles and you want to spend less, the Wilkinet (£28.95), available by mail order on 01239 831246, is for you. It relies on being tied correctly.

Easiest to find is the Tomy Cradle Carrier (£29.99). Both Boots and Mothercare sell it. You must try this properly before you buy it as it is not for everyone.

Car Seats

There are many models of seats and even more models of cars, and some cannot be used together safely. A survey by the BSI uncovered some disturbing safety blunders: two-thirds of the five thousand seats surveyed were incorrectly fitted, and 50 per cent of children were not strapped in properly.

The most important things to remember are:
- Ignore your friends' advice unless their car is identical to yours.
- Try before you buy: each make and model of car varies in

seatbelt length and position as well as car-seat shape, and this will affect how the child restraint fits.
- Buy a baby seat before the baby is born if she is being driven home from hospital. Do not hold a baby on your lap or put a seatbelt round both of you. In an accident, the baby could be crushed.

The best place to buy a car seat is a specialist nursery store or even a specialist car-seat retailer such as the Milton Keynes In-Car Safety Centre, tel. 01908 220909. Our star buys in this section are available at virtually all good independent retailers, as well as the Early Learning Centre, Mothercare and Children's World.

Mirrors that attach to your own rear-view mirror allow you to watch what's going on in the back seat and are available from most nursery retailers. The Child View Mirror by First Years is available from the Early Learning Centre, at £3.99.

Child In-Car Care

The RMI (Retail Motor Industry Federation), in partnership with the Child Accident Prevention Trust, approved dealers and local authorities run a Fit Safe Sit Safe – Child In-Car Care Scheme. This offers free advice and information on caring for the safety of children in cars. They help and advise with selecting and fitting suitable car seats for your particular make of car. It is a good idea to seek advice from them *before* buying your seat.

For a list of recognized RMI centres in your area, contact the road safety officer at one of the following local authorities:

Cambridgeshire: 01223 317385; Cheshire: 01244 603728; Cleveland: 01642 262690; City of Coventry: 01203 832023; Derbyshire: 01629 580202; Devon: 01392 383216; East Sussex: 01273 482303; Essex: 01245 492211; Hereford and Worcester: 01684 893232; Hertfordshire: 01992 556098; Leicestershire: 01162 657227; Northamptonshire: 01604 763438; Oxfordshire: 01865 815657; Stockport: 0161 474

4876; Suffolk: (Ipswich) 01473 265621, (Lowestoft) 01502 562262; Warwickshire: 01926 412251.

Over the next two years, more local authorities in the UK will be participating.

The law and car seats

- Children under three travelling in the front seat of a car must use an approved restraint suited to their age and weight.
- The driver is responsible for children under fourteen wearing a seatbelt.
- Adult passengers and drivers must wear a seatbelt if one is available.

In-car dangers

- Watch your child's fingers if you have electric windows.
- Never leave your child alone in the car. Car theft is at an all-time high and it may be incidental to a thief that your child is strapped in a car seat in the back. A sleeping baby is at risk of carbon monoxide poisoning if left in a car with the engine running.
- Summer heat can kill. Temperatures inside a car on a hot day are much higher than those outside. Your child will suffer rapid dehydration in a stationary car.
- Cover car seats if you have to park in the heat. The metal parts will get so hot they could burn your baby.

Safety check – car travel with a baby

- Get used to fitting the seatbelt round the infant-carrier exactly as recommended. In an accident, a poorly fitted seatbelt will offer little or no protection.
- Check that the baby's harness is secured: the seatbelt anchors the carrier, not the baby.
- Always adjust the harness according to the thickness of the baby's clothing.

- Additional head support such as a head-hugger is recommended for the baby's first three months. Some seats have one included in the price, but you may have to buy one separately.
- Ensure that the carrier is not in its rocking position when you fit it in the car.
- When your baby's head sticks up above the top of the car seat, he has outgrown it.

!!!
* If your car has a passenger airbag, do not use the front seat for your baby or child.
* Never tuck blankets or cushions into a child's car seat, or use cushions or a towel to raise the chair so that your baby can see out the window. It affects safety in a crash.

Harnesses

Child seats with five-point harnesses are the safest. Ensure that two straps go over the child's shoulders and two fit round the legs. The fifth strap is designed to pass between the legs, preventing the child from sliding out of the seat on impact.

The shoulder straps should pass through the child seat at shoulder height, to be raised as the child grows. Crotch straps should be kept short – just one inch of slack can dramatically increase the force on a child in an accident. Once she is strapped in, the harness should be tightened as much as possible. You should be able to fit two fingers only between the belt and the child's chest. Replace the seat if the webbing is frayed or the buckles do not do up and undo smoothly.

If the child seat has been in an accident you must replace it, even if you cannot see any damage. The belt or buckle mechanism could have been damaged.

Getting Around

Second-Hand Car Seats

More than a third of all car seats in use are second-hand, but unless you know the chair's full history you cannot be sure that it has not been involved in an accident. So never buy a car seat through a second-hand shop, car boot sale or an advertisement.

Also be wary of a chair that does not have a full set of fitting instructions.

Rental Bargains

Kwik-Fit hire out fitted car seats for £39.90. A new seat is used for each rental, and you keep the seat until your child is four. If you return it in good condition you will get a £20 refund in Kwik-Fit vouchers. Telephone 0131 337 9200 for details.

Some county councils run a baby rent-a-seat system whereby you can hire a seat for as long as you need it. Contact the road safety officer at your local council to see if they have this scheme. Leeds Rent-a-seat have details of council hire in Yorkshire (0113 246 1773).

Carrycots with Restraints

Restraints are designed to tether the carrycot but not the baby inside. They are therefore not safe as your baby could be thrown out. If you have to use one, ensure that your baby is also wearing a five-point harness.

Stage 1 Baby Seats

Baby seats for newborns up to 22lb may appear to be a short-term investment, but they are hugely popular. Although it is safe for a baby to go straight into a Stage 1 and 2 combined seat, many parents are concerned that a tiny child might feel 'lost' in a larger chair. The stage 1 seats provide excellent support for the baby and are easy to handle as they use adult lap belts as a fastening. They can also be used in the home, making it possible to lift the baby in and out of the car without disturbing her. Whenever she is in the seat, the harness should be used. Some seats come with a head-hugger, but you may need to buy one separately. A rigid handle is best as seats are designed to be carried in the crook of your arm. Your back and tummy may feel weak for a while after the birth so good posture is important. Expect to pay £30 to £45.

What to look for

- **The fit.** If the seatbelt is too tight, the carrier will be tilted too upright to hold your baby safely and comfortably.
- **Weight.** Ensure that the seat is easy to carry and is not too heavy. Try lifting it with something weighing around 10kg in the seat.
- **Special features.** Look out for reclining and rocking positions, nappy compartments and bottle-holders. Some seats include storage compartments and hooks to fit on to shopping trolleys.
- **Cleaning.** A machine-washable cover is essential.
- **Adjustability.** Ensure that the harness is easy for you to adjust, but not so easy for the baby.
- **Compatibility.** Some car manufacturers specify their preferred car seats.
- **Padding.** Too little will be uncomfortable for your baby on a long ride.

★★★ Star buys ★★★

Consider the following: Britax Rock-a-Bye (£44.99); Klippan Carry Tot (£42, including head-hugger), which can be used as a rocking-chair; Klippan Carry Tot Royale (£46, including head-hugger), which has a compartment in the back of the seat. Similar models to the Klippan ones can be found under the Mothercare own-brand label. The Britax Rock-a-Tot will be in the shops in 1996.

For parents of multiples or those with weak backs, a spacious, light seat is the Maxi Cosi 1500. This weighs only 1.9kg, as opposed to the 2.5kg Carry Tot or the 3.4kg Rock-a-Bye, though it is more expensive. It is available at independent nursery stores at around £49.99.

Cumfi's Swing 'n' Go is worth considering if you have the space and the money (£99). This is a car seat that fits on to a swing frame, so at home you can hang the baby in the frame where she is rocked quietly to sleep (if you are lucky).

Stage 1 and 2 Combined Seats

These seats are suitable for children from birth to around four. They face the rear until the baby is nine months old, when they can be adjusted to face the front. They are good value for money at £43 to £100. The seats are difficult to move from car to car, so ensure that you are happy about fixing them in place.

What to look for

- **Fit.** If it only fits one way in your car it is of little use.
- **Straps.** These can be tricky to fit as there are more of them than most seats have.
- **Harness.** Bear in mind that you will have to adjust this on every trip. You need something simple and efficient.
- **Height.** Make sure that the seat is high enough to enable your baby to look outside.

★★★ Star buy ★★★

The Klippan Easirider, £39.99, is great value for a sturdy seat.

Stage 2 Seats

These are forward-facing seats for babies over six months and up to four years. They are well padded with a high back.

What to look for

Look for the same features as with stage-1-and-2 combined seats, plus:
- The reclining mechanism should be attached to the front of the seat so that you can recline the chair without having to get out of your seat to operate it.
- Some models take play trays, which both entertain and act as an extra measure to stop the baby trying to get out of the seat.

★★★ Star buys ★★★

The Freeway XL (£84) converts from upright to a reclining position. It is easy to adjust and not too massive.

The Bébé Confort Cosmos (£99.99) is worth considering if you are not buying a baby carrier. You can buy a Newly Born Kit cushion for £5.99 with the seat to give your baby extra support.

Stage 2 and 3 Combined Seats

These are the most convenient car seats for people with more than one car. Expect to pay £50 to £100.
- They can be moved in and out of the car in seconds.
- An adult lap and shoulder belt fastens the seat in place. No extra fixings are required.
- They are light, often made of moulded polystyrene and little else.
- They last from six months to around six years old, depending on the model you choose.

★★★ Star buy ★★★

Britax Super Cruiser (£49). This seat is extremely light and can easily be transferred from one car to another. If your baby will frequently be driven around in various cars, this is the one for you.

Prams and Buggies

> *'What often happens is a man rushes into the department, waves a pram catalogue under my nose and says, "She'll have that one." I say, "Don't you want to see how it works and discuss whether it is suitable for your lifestyle?" And he says, "That's the one she likes the look of, so that's the one she's getting."'*
>
> **Sales assistant, Swindon**

Only buy a pram if you intend to do some serious walking in town and your baby needs support and protection for hours at a time. Good suspension is as important in city streets as in country lanes. If you do most of your travelling by car and will only be taking your baby out to go to the park or to sit in the garden, a pram is not necessary. The most versatile conveyance is the fully reclining buggy or pushchair. These can be up to £200 cheaper than many prams, do a good job and can be easily slipped into a car boot.

Look at the full range of models and decide which one suits your budget and your own needs. For example, can it be collapsed easily to fit into the boot of your car and leave room for other items? If you are looking at a combination pram/pushchair, remember that it will be used as a pushchair for far longer than as a pram, so always choose the type of pushchair you like before considering carrycot options.

Before going to the shops, look in the second-hand section of your local paper. Maclaren and Silver Cross prams and buggies are built to last and you may find a bargain. If you are buying a second-hand carrycot, check carefully that the fabric is clean, aired and rot-free. Always buy a new mattress.

Buying a pram is the infant equivalent of buying a car. The general types of prams and pushchairs are:
- a traditional pram;

- a convertible model, where the seat adapts from carrycot into pushchair;
- pushchair or buggy – some models can recline fully, making them suitable for newborn babies.

Always:
- Use your buggy for the number of children for which it was built – one per seat.
- Use the brakes, even when stopping briefly.
- Use a safety harness. Some nasty accidents are caused by babies falling out of prams.
- Make sure all safety catches click into place before you use it.
- Keep your conveyance well maintained. Most pram and buggy suppliers sell lubricant for the wheels.
- If parts start to wear, ensure that the pram or buggy is serviced by a reputable repair-centre.

Never:
- Hang shopping bags over buggy handles. It can cause them to tip.
- Leave a dog tied to a pram or pushchair.
- Let a child play on it. The stability may not support his weight.
- Open or close parts of a pram or buggy without checking that your baby's fingers are out of the way.

Hiring

You can hire a buggy or pram for around £70 for six months. Contact the Baby Equipment Hirers Association on 0113 278 5560 for details of local agents.

Look out for the new Cosatto Swallow prams and pushchairs, which come with an easy-fold chassis. This has lockable swivel wheels for easy manoeuvrability and does just what its name suggests – and needs only one hand. Simply push and squeeze the handle, push the bar with your foot and the frame collapses into a compact fold. To open, just depress the footbar and pull the handle.

Prams

Traditional Carriage Prams

These are hard-wearing with a solid body and large wheels.

> **PLUS POINTS**
> * They offer the baby tremendous comfort and protection.
> * When the baby is older, he can sit up in the pram with a harness on.
> * The suspension and handling are superb.
>
> **MINUS POINTS**
> * They are not suitable for car-users as it is often complicated to dismantle them.
> * If you have to negotiate stairs or steps, they are difficult to manoeuvre.
> * They take up a lot of room.

Any nanny worth her salt will tell you that there is only one make to buy, and that is Silver Cross. Prices range from £205 for the Bilbao to £475 for the Marlborough or Silver Stream. John Lewis also stocks scaled-down toy versions of these for children, £169 for the Royal. Stalk Talk has special offers on discontinued colours. (Tel. 0115 930 6700 or fax 0115 930 4700 for details.) Your goods will be delivered to the door and you can order by phone using Access or Visa.

If you have only a vague idea of what you are looking for, ring Silver Cross for brochures to help you make a decision. Before placing your order, you might be able to try out your preferred options in a local nursery shop. You do not want to be lumbered with a model that is too heavy.

If you are going to be pushing your pram around after dark, NCT Sales (tel. 0141 633 5552) sell a luminous reflector strip to fit round the hood, price £4.

If you have a carriage pram that has been in your family for generations and needs restoration, inquire at your local shops.

If they cannot help, you will find specialist restoration skills and a stock of original parts for old models at Harold Stewart's, 64 Stockport Road, Ardwick, Manchester, tel. 0161 273 5861.

Convertibles/Two-in-Ones

These prams convert from a fully reclining pram into a pushchair by folding or removing part of the carrycot.

PLUS POINTS
* They take up the least space of the three pram options.
* They can be very robust, with good suspension.
* They can be stored in most reasonably sized car boots.

MINUS POINTS
* There is no carrycot you can take on and off the chassis with the baby inside.
* Unlike a carrycot, the lie-flat option is not suitable for use as a baby's first bed.
* The baby can slide out if not properly restrained.
* They can be bulky, and may not fit into smaller car boots.

★★★ Star buys ★★★

For style, look at Mamas & Papas Ciao (£229) and the Carisma (£359); an efficient model is the Maclaren Clio (£199.99). All of these can be seen at Children's World.

Check out the following brands:

Bébé Confort (telephone 01732 740880 for a catalogue), Cossatto Swallow (telephone 01268 727070 for a catalogue).

The Two-in-One Plus

This is more or less the same as a two-in-one, except that when the seat is reclined flat like a carrycot, it can be lifted in and out of the chassis. However, you still cannot use this as a bed. These prams can be heavy, bulky and difficult to store, but if you do not have a car and are intending to wheel your pram/pushchair out of your hall and into the street, this probably will not matter.

★★★ Star buys ★★★

The Mothercare Super Italia (£299) has a continental flavour and looks as if it should cost twice as much. All prams and pushchairs or buggies from Mothercare come with a twelve-month guarantee.

The Maclaren Chantelle, at £279, is due out in 1996 and is well worth a test drive, as is their Sorrento XL (£329), which offers sensational suspension. One of Maclaren's many plus points is that they are based in Britain. If you have a problem or need a spare, the chances are it can be sorted out in days rather than the weeks needed by some continental manufacturers.

Three-in-Ones

These consist of a chassis on to which you fix a carrycot (which can double as the baby's bed as well) or pushchair seat.

PLUS POINTS
* This is often the most economical buy as you can dispense with a separate carrycot or crib.
* It is useful if you have a lot of stairs which you would rather not negotiate with the pram.
* Some fold down to fit the smallest car boots.

MINUS POINTS
* The cheaper models have no springs, which means a rough ride for the baby.
* They can be complicated to put together.

If you can afford £215 for a pushchair and £187 for an optional carrycot, Bébécar products such as the Limousine and Turbo 02 offer numerous well-designed features including adaptable handle heights, good-sized shopping basket and excellent suspension.

The classic gift from mothers-in-law is a Silver Cross three-in-one. If money is no object, she may be interested in the Ultima and Carriba, due in the shops in 1996.

Just to confuse you, Mamas & Papas produce four-in-ones, so-called because they combine a pram, carrycot, pushchair and foot rest. Models include Classic Chic (£465.99) and Babychic (£409). The Mamas & Papas brochure is obtainable by calling 01484 4382222. The name Five-in-One has been invented by Silver Cross to describe a chassis with three interchangeable pieces of equipment – a car seat, carrycot, and pushchair seat attachment. The car seat can also be used as a mini-pushchair seat. Models available are the Arriva (£410) and the Astora (£345). To compound the confusion, without the car seat, the manufacturers refer to this as a three-in-one. The Maclaren Superdreamer costs £250 and offers a similar package.

Pushchairs and Buggies

Broadly speaking, most people consider a pushchair to be a larger, bulkier chair attached to a chassis. A buggy, on the other hand, can either 'umbrella' fold like a bunch of sticks, or fold flat to occupy minimal space. However, there is a fine line between these definitions and some bulkier chairs fold into remarkably small packages.

For a single baby, choose a fully reclining pushchair or an umbrella-folding type. If you are having trouble attaching a stroller bag to your buggy, cable ties will hold it securely in place. Any DIY enthusiast or electrician will be able to give you some. They will cost a few pence from electrical retailers.

The Fully Reclining Pushchair

These have a seat which reclines to a virtually horizontal position (some models have carrycots and car seats which fit on to the same chassis). Look out for integral shower hoods or sun canopies.

> **PLUS POINTS**
> * They can be used from birth.
> * Many have sprung suspension.
> * Most have trays for shopping.
>
> **MINUS POINTS**
> * Seat units have little padding and do not give the baby much protection, though you can buy an insert for around £9.99.
> * They can be very bulky when folded up.
> * Those with swivel wheels can be rather unstable on bumpy ground, but they can be locked in place.

The Cumfi Mirage at £99.99 is excellent value, but its swivel wheels are not lockable. This does not matter to everyone. If it matters to you, look out for the Mothercare Seville (£169). Although it is not as nippy, it has a range of additional features, such as adjustable handle height, lockable wheels and a 'flip-over' handle, so that you can have your baby facing you as you walk.

Also worth looking out for is the Maclaren Melody Deluxe (£149), which has the advantage of being an umbrella-folding type. It does not have a shopping tray, so you will have to buy a stroller bag (Clippasafe, available at £5.99 at Children's World and most nursery-equipment retailers). The Swallow Top de Luxe (£180) is a similar model.

Mountain/All-Terrain Buggies

For those who want to enjoy the beach and the countryside with their baby. These are by necessity heavy and sturdy.

There is a choice of two brands: the Mountain Buggy, which has special 'packages' for newborns, twins and special needs children, and PCD's Rover range of all-terrain pushchairs. They are all well-made products. As there may well be changes in the design of the Mountain Buggy during 1996, the sensible thing would be to send off for both leaflets. The main differences at present are in weight, fabrics, closing mechanism, wheel sizes and suitability for newborns. The Mountain Buggy comes with a sun hood, storm cover and gear tray included in the price; with PCD you buy these separately.

Both companies can be contacted by phone or fax, Mountain Buggy (UK) on 0181 747 9439, PCD on 01823 491026.

The Maclaren/Umbrella-Fold

This is a lightweight buggy which folds up like an umbrella and normally weighs less than the baby.

PLUS POINTS
* Cheap.
* Easy to use.
* Easy to store.
* Excellent for use on public transport.

MINUS POINTS
* Should not be used until the baby can sit up (at around six months).
* The folding mechanism leaves nowhere to put shopping.
* They are easily distorted if you try to fold them wrongly.

Other models worth considering are the Plikomatic by Mamas & Papas, £168. If you intend to travel extensively with your baby, the Bébécar Laser (£129) is an excellent buy. Its compact folded size means it is usually allowed into aeroplanes as hand luggage and has a roomy seat that will be comfortable for toddlers as well as babies.

British buyers tend to dislike the fixed front wheels, but if you buy this buggy in Europe (where it does not have to conform to British Safety Standards) you should be able to find a swivel-wheeled version.

If you want a second buggy simply to keep in the car or for a holiday, the following all cost £29.99 and are suitable for use from six months: Maclaren Imp (from the Early Learning

Centre), Mothercare Basic and the Quest Stroller (from Children's World).

For features such as lockable swivel wheels and a seat with more than one position, expect to pay up to £90.

The Chicco three-position stroller (£69.99) is widely available. It has a three-position lie-back seat unit, lockable swivel front wheels and an adjustable leg rest.

Buggies for Two or More Babies

There are two types, twin buggies and tandems. Both have their good and bad points. You must try pushing them around fully loaded before making a decision, making sure you test them round corners and up steps. It is normally weight that sways most people.

The Twin

In this type the babies sit side by side.

PLUS POINTS
* They go up and down kerbs easily.
* Two children can sit reclined in comfort.
* It is easy to see both children.
* They tend to be light.
* They often fold down to a small size.

MINUS POINTS
* They are awkward in shops and at supermarket checkouts.
* Only some models fit through standard doorways.
* Children can lean over and fight with each other.
* A wide-awake child can disturb a sleeping one.
* There may be nowhere to put your shopping.
* They can strain your back.

The Maclaren Duette for £179 is excellent. Remember that pushing around two children is heavy work and this model is lightweight, durable and suitable for babies from birth. Buggylovers everywhere are waiting with bated breath for the launch of the Twin Mirage by Cumfi, which may happen towards the end of 1996. It will cost around £170, including hoods and a single apron.

The Tandem

In this version one baby sits behind the other.

PLUS POINTS
* They are slim, so you can go everywhere a single buggy can go.
* An older child in front can chat to you while the baby sleeps behind.
* Most have capacious shopping trays.

MINUS POINTS
* They can be heavy and difficult to push up kerbs or steps.
* They are often bulky when folded up.
* There can be fights over who has the front seat.

The Cumfi Twingo at £165 is extremely good value. It comes complete with a PVC storm cover and has a padded handle that makes a huge difference when you are trying to manoeuvre it. The Waki Rider GTi (£200 including rain cover) was also singled out by our testers for its adjustable handle and good-sized seats. This model is better for transporting a baby and a toddler than twins.

Waki also make the Bertie (£139.99), a light buggy, suitable for use from six months. This has a platform on the back, behind the baby's pushchair, on which an older child can stand. If no one is standing on the platform you can unfold a huge shopping bag to sit there instead. Waki have just developed a model that is suitable for newborn use. This should be available in 1996.

Twins and Multiples

Unless you need a particularly rugged pram, go for a light, durable one. Mamas & Papas make the enticing Micro, but obtaining this model may involve an extremely long delivery time, and because they are based in Italy, parts and repairs are not as straightforward as they are with British-made goods.

The Maclaren Duette (see page 282), a side-by-side, lightweight umbrella-fold chair 74cm wide and weighing 10kg, is great for twins. You may be able to buy one second-hand from your twins club as older babies progress to the Maclaren Twin Tourer, the lightest buggy we could find (£150).

Most tandems are not designed for two children of a similar age but for an older sibling and a baby. Be sure to check before you buy. The Bébécar Dupla (£329), and the Cumfifolda Twingo (£165) are both intended for twins. Also see Mountain-buggy, above.

If you live near Nottingham and you are expecting twins or more, Nippers at Hall Farm, Flawborough, tel. 01949 851244 is wonderful. Not only will you get a discount, but you can delight in the knowledge that Emma Hawthorne and her staff will bust a gut to find products that really suit you.

Triplets

When triplets are tiny, you may have to fit all three into a twin buggy. Make sure that you can install the appropriate restraints. If you do not want to put all three in a twin, you can always carry one baby in a sling. There are two suppliers of buggies for triplets and quads in the UK: Petrena Products, tel. 0116 2605966, and Gordons Prams, tel. 0161 834 4600, a shop in Manchester that makes and sells quad pushchairs.

If in doubt:
- Get the 12-page leaflet *Guide to Pushchairs and Car Seats for Twins, Triplets and Quads*, £2 from TAMBA, tel. 0151 348 0020. This gives the makes, dimensions and addresses of the manufacturers. Enclose an SAE.
- Find out about second-hand models from the TAMBA administrator.

You might telephone the following manufacturers for their catalogues.

Bébécar UK, tel. 0181 201 0505. Their triplet buggy should be available in the UK soon, but it might not feature in the current catalogue.

Emmaljunga, tel. 0116 260 5966.

Maclaren, tel. 01327 842662.

Mamas & Papas, tel. 01484 431758.

Accessories

Buy all the accessories you want at the same time as you buy your pram or buggy, because many companies alter colours and patterns at regular intervals and you may be unable to match them if you wait. You will also be fully prepared for the British weather at the outset. If you delay until you really need your canopy or rain cover, the chances are that it will be out of stock. In some cases, accessories are included in the cost of the pram or buggy.

Sunshades

Do not buy a parasol as they need frequent adjustment and can be quite delicate. A canopy costing around £15 offers proper protection from the sun.

Rain covers

A set of waterproof covers for your pushchair (around £16) will protect your baby from bad weather. They often have to be removed before you fold up the pushchair.

If you don't want to wheel mud into the house, put a showercap on each pram wheel before you go indoors. The ones you get free in hotel bathrooms are ideal.

Harnesses

To be safe in a pushchair, your baby needs to be held in place with a five-point harness which goes over both shoulders, across the waist and between the legs. If it is not supplied as standard on your pushchair, buy one separately. All models have rings to fasten the harness to the seat. Harnesses cost between £5 and £10, depending on whether they are made of webbing or leather.

Carrycot Covers

Carrycots tend not to be waterproof, so you will probably need a waterproof cover, which costs around £14, especially if you are also using the carrycot indoors as the baby's bed.

Buggy Liners

These provide padding to keep a newborn baby comfortable in a fully reclining buggy seat. They cost around £10.

Muffs and Cosytoes

These are like infant sleeping bags and prevent the baby from getting cold. Bear in mind that they are only needed in the most severe weather conditions, and take care not to let your baby overheat. They cost around £20.

Protective Nets

If you leave your baby out in the garden in the pram, you may wish to buy either a cat net or an insect net to protect his face. The mesh on an insect net is finer, for obvious reasons.

The Lock-away Locking Device

Useful if you want to secure your pram or buggy to an immovable object while you go into a shop. This locking device extends over 1.5m and costs £9.50. Call 01222 464463 for stockists.

Shopping Trays or Nets

These often come as part of the pram or buggy. If not, it is a good idea to invest in one if your model has space to accommodate it.

Bedding

It is a waste of money to buy sheets for the cot *and* the pram. Instead use your cot sheets folded to fit the pram. Old pillowcases can be converted into pram quilts or double-sided covers for the pram mattress. You can also cut down your own old sheets for the baby.

Buying second-hand

If the pram or pushchair is more than five years old, you may have problems finding parts. Check that:

- All foldings parts move smoothly without catching anywhere.
- Both the primary and secondary locks work well so that the pushchair cannot close up with your child in it.
- The brakes are in good working order, and strong enough to hold the pram or buggy still even if you push quite hard.
- The seat fabric is not torn. Tears make cleaning difficult and could be a hazard.
- The wheels are not worn in odd places. This could weaken the frame.
- The wheels are touching the ground equally. If they do not, the frame is probably bent.
- The buggy is not rusty.
- Ideally, the instructions are with it.

Cycling with a Baby

Your baby should be able to sit up on his own before you put him in a child seat on a bicycle. Some people cycle with smaller babies in a sling, but this is not a good idea as it affects your balance.

Ensure that your bicycle is suitable.
- Is it in good condition?
- Does it brake efficiently?
- Is the frame strong?
- Can you tackle steep hills with ease?

Safety

Most injuries involving children in child seats occur when their feet get caught in the spokes of the wheel. Never use a seat without some sort of shield between the child's feet and the wheel. Remember:
- A harness is essential.
- There is no British standard for child cycle seats, so you will have to use your common sense to judge how robust it is.
- Check that the seat has a full set of instructions. If you cannot understand them, ask your cycle shop to fit the seat for you.
- Some seats rust, especially round the brackets and bolts that hold them together. This can lead to them breaking while in use, so go for a seat which has sturdy joints made from something more weather-resistant than painted steel.
- Dress brightly if you are cycling in traffic or during darker times of day.

Front-Mounted Seats

RoSPA (the Royal Society for the Prevention of Accidents believes that accidents are much more likely with seats which are mounted over the handlebars and/or front wheel, for the following reasons:
- They may affect steering and balance.
- The child (and sometimes the seat, too) might be flung forward when the rider brakes.

- The rider's vision can be interrupted or distracted by having a child in front because she rides in a peculiar position to compensate for the additional weight.
- Many models lack harnesses – a major safety drawback.

Back-Mounted Seats

Before you look at these, RoSPA suggest that you check your bike. Make sure that it can take the weight of a seat and a child (many can't), and that the fixing brackets on the seat are compatible with the carrier tubes. If you are going to carry luggage as well as your baby, change your back-mounted storage boxes for 'low riders' at the front – this will balance the load and improve the bike's stability. The more brackets that fasten the seat to the bike, the better. Brackets should be robust. Good features to look for are:
- a high back;
- foot and hand rests;
- side protection;
- a light weight;
- a three-point harness (one that goes over each shoulder to meet one from the crotch).

Adult tricycles with child seats already installed are available from W. R. Pashley Ltd, tel. 01789 292263, at around £569. Pashley's child seats for tricycles can be ordered through your local bike shop.

★★★ Star buys ★★★

The Discovery series from HAMAX costs between £59.99 and £79.99. Fischer of Finchley, tel. 0181 805 3088, distribute these in the UK.

If you want to be able to switch the baby seat easily from your bicycle to your partner's, look out for Rhode Gear. Instead of bolting the seat on to the bike, you clip it on to a pannier rack which is included in the cost of the baby seat. You can buy an extra rack for £34.99 to fit any other bike that may be used to transport your baby. The Rhode Gear Taxi costs £69.99; the Rhode Gear Limo, £99.99, converts to a baby chair off the bike. For stockists call the importers Madison Cycles plc on 0181 954 5421.

Babywear for Bicycling

In winter, wrap up your baby as warmly as you dare. Remember to take precautions against sunburn in the summer.

Cycling Helmets

Head protection is essential. Try the helmet on the child before you buy it. It must meet one of the following standards: BS6863 1989, ANSI Z90.4, SNELL B90 or AS 2063.86. The helmet is a good fit if it is:
- snug with the straps adjusted;
- unable to move backwards, forwards or from side to side;
- comfortable and does not obstruct vision;
- not covering your baby's ears;
- well ventilated to allow a flow of cool air, especially to the forehead.

*** **Star buy** ***

The HAMAX Up-to-3 (£27.95) offers maximum protection and low weight.

16 Travel

When planning your holiday, consider the following – unless you are the adventurous sort who relishes the idea of backpacking with a baby on board.
- Choose somewhere where young families are welcomed rather than barely tolerated.
- You will need good local shops if you are preparing baby foods and require access to washing facilities, nappies, a pharmacy etc.
- Places with lots of steps, stairs or steep hills should be avoided if you are going to be without a car and using a buggy.
- If you want to eat *à deux* at night you will need to inquire about baby-listening and babysitting services, and be sure to take your monitor.
- You do not want to be dependent on someone else's rickety cot. These can be lethal. If in doubt, hire one for the holiday.
- If your baby is crawling, take some table corners, string and scissors so that you can make your room as safe as possible.
- Will you have access to a launderette or washing service?

Make sure that you put your baby on your passport or she will not be able to leave Great Britain or enter another country. It is possible to register the baby on both your own and your partner's passport if you think she will need to travel with one parent only on occasions.

You need to send off Renewal Passport Form C (available

from a main post office) with the baby's original birth or adoption certificate and the relevant passport. This costs £5 and takes a minimum of two weeks.

Alternatively, for £18 the baby can have her own passport. The photograph will have to be renewed every five years, either at the passport office or by post, until the bearer is sixteen years old and eligible for an adult passport.

There is bound to be a point while you are travelling where you have to carry everything in one go, so make sure that your essentials – money, passports etc. – are easily accessible to you but not to a pickpocket. Some people adopt the Big-Bag technique, keeping essentials along with nappies in a changing bag. Others prefer to keep travel documents on their person zipped up in a bum bag.

Equipment

If you are only going away for a couple of weeks, be absolutely sure that everything you take is necessary. Can you pack it easily? Remember that there is a limit to how much you can carry, especially when there is a baby as well. If you are buying equipment especially for the holiday, will it be of use afterwards?

Lightweight Buggies

If you are borrowing or hiring one:
- It must be an umbrella-folding type if you are going to be using public transport.
- Check that you can open and close it one-handed with your baby tucked under your arm.
- The best type lock shut automatically.

Travel Cots

If you are concerned that a sturdy cot will not be available at your destination, hire one for the trip. These are worth buying only if:

- You spend a lot of time in the kitchen at home – a travel cot can double as a playpen.
- A friend or relative frequently looks after your baby and would appreciate a travel cot at his or her house.
- You can find a friend or relative to share the cost and use of it. When neither of you no longer need it, you might be able to sell it and recoup some of the cost.

★★★ Star buys ★★★

Travel Lite, £79.99 and the Petite Star travel cot at £69.99, from independent retailers, are great value. Both of these are hard-wearing and extremely easy to erect and fold away, and both include carrying cases.

The Cumfi Travel Lite Sport (£99) comes complete with insect net, toy bag and mattress cover.

Sterilizing Equipment

If you are taking your steam sterilizer, make sure that you have the necessary adaptor to plug it in at your destination. If you don't want to be burdened with such a bulky object, you can buy DSB disposable sterilizing bags (£5.50 for seven days' supply) from John Lewis stores. These bags can simply be hung from a tap in the bathroom while sterilizing bottles and bits.

Otherwise, the most compact steam sterilizer is the Babytec 'Home & Away' sterilizer. It measures five inches high when stored and can sterilize two standard-shaped bottles in eight minutes. £24.99 from the Great Little Trading Company mail order, tel. 0171 376 3337.

Desperation

If your baby is very noisy and active and you are dreading the journey, discuss the options available with your GP. He may suggest prescribing a mild sedative for your baby. But this option is not suitable for a very small baby.

Packing checklist

Bottles	Swimming gear
Formula	Monitor
Sterilizer (electric or other)	Changing bag
Bottle brush	Travel cot and bedding
Buggy and canopy	Toys and comforter
Sling or backpack	Cool bag for bottles and baby food
Bibs	
T-shirts and sun hat	Baby food
Waterproof sunblock	Equipment for expressing milk if required
Wipes	
Nappy sacks	First-aid kit
Barrier cream	Mosquito repellent for babies
Clothes	

Air Travel

When you pack your hand luggage, anticipate a delay. Gatwick Airport has had to help numerous mothers who have checked in their luggage complete with formula, medicines, nappies and toys which they suddenly, and urgently, need. Keep your buggy as hand luggage until you board the plane. The cabin crew will take it and it will be returned to you in the baggage hall.

Children under two travelling on a parent's lap will be charged the infant fare, which is 10 per cent of the adult fare, on most international flights. Within the UK they are carried free.

British Airways suggest that when you book your flight you should:

- Request bulkhead seats. These have extra leg-room and preference will be given to mothers with babies if they are available.
- Book a bassinet or sky cot if you are travelling on a long-haul flight.
- Ask for pre-boarding when you arrive in the departure lounge.

British Airways and many other long-haul airlines have a dedicated crew member responsible for giving extra assistance to mothers with babies. They will provide nappies, baby food and bottles and warm up baby milk on request.

Newer long-haul aeroplanes have baby changing facilities in the toilets.

Breast or bottle feeding the baby on take-off and landing should help prevent pain in the ears caused by the change in cabin pressure.

Car Seats on Planes

If you are paying the appropriate fare for a child aged between six months and three years to occupy a seat, you can take a suitable children's car seat on board. This can be placed on the seat next to the parent. Car seats must conform to the following criteria:

- They must be purpose-designed for air travel.
- They must be in good condition and not show any obvious signs of having sustained damage.

Your seat will be suitable only if it can be restrained by a lap belt.

Car Travel

What to take in the car

- Cassette with songs.
- Toys and your baby's comforter.
- Cool bag with bottles/snacks if required.
- First-aid kit.

A clip-on play tray is quite a good idea for the more active infant on a long journey. These are made to fit on to most car seats. Without one, the person sitting in the front passenger seat will find him or herself leaning backwards to scrabble on the floor for an endless cascade of cloth books, rattles and teethers. These trays are not foolproof, however: there are bound to be several missiles launched from the tray that end up somewhere unreachable.

Remember that your baby's car seat might come in useful at your destination.

Coach Travel

On a coach you cannot take all the gear you can fit into a car, but at least you can give your baby your total attention. Remember that it will be virtually impossible to get to your luggage during the journey. Keep with you even more toys and books than you would in the car, and a coat or cover-up so that you can take your baby out for a breather at each stop.

Ferries

There are often good changing and feeding facilities on ferries.

For long crossings, hire a cabin so that you and your baby have a quiet base. Sometimes travel cots are available – ask when you book. Do not leave your buggy in the car – you can usually wheel it round the deck.

Train Travel

As the toilet facilities on trains are unreliable you would be well advised to take extra wipes and a change of clothes.

PART NINE
FASHION, FUN AND GAMES

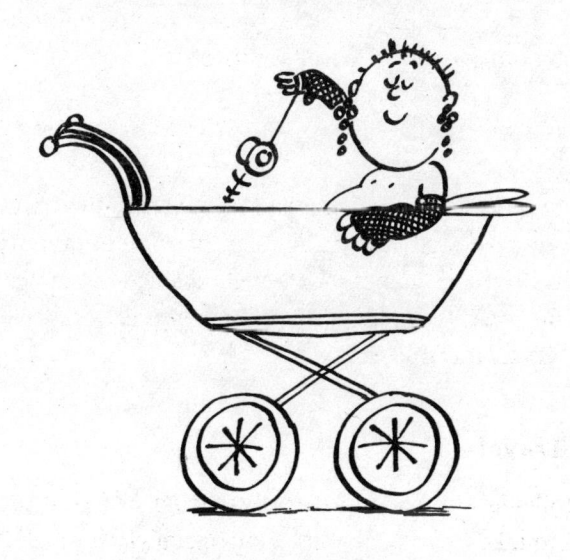

17 Dressing

Baby Clothes

There are so many enchanting little outfits pleading to be bought that should you feel a 'splurge' coming on, don't forget the following:
- If your baby is not yet born, you will not know his exact size until he appears.
- Buy clothes on the large side. If he is three months old, buy a six-month size – babies grow out of their clothes in a few weeks. In addition, so much wear and washing tends to make baby clothes shrink a little.
- Look for pale colours. Regurgitated milk destroys navy blue in an instant.
- Avoid hand-wash-only items.
- If you are buying from a market stall or are given a home-made item, check it very carefully to ensure that there are no pins or needles left inside by accident.

To check your baby's weight, weigh yourself on the bathroom scales, then pick up your baby, weigh both of you together and subtract your own weight from the joint weight.

What to look for
- Choose natural fabrics which allow the baby's skin to breathe and minimize allergic reactions.
- Check that buttons and fastenings are strongly attached. Oversew them if necessary.

- Avoid clothes with a long seam down the back. Your baby spends so much time lying on it that he could be very uncomfortable.
- Feel inside clothes to check how the seams are finished. Are they likely to rub against his skin?

Cut in half any looped tags such as washing-instruction labels. You could inadvertently catch a little finger inside them during a change. They can also cause irritation.

Sleepsuits and Babygros

These are standard issue for the contemporary baby and can be worn during the day and at night. Most are made from stretch terry towelling or a cotton and polyester mix. Look for glove attachments if your newborn is prone to scratching his face with his nails. Scratch mitts tend to fall off.

Avoid back-fastening suits as they are tricky to manage and uncomfortable for the baby when he lies on his back. The best stretchsuit has poppers down the front and down one or both legs to allow easy nappy changing – you don't want to be slipping pooey babygros over your baby's face.

If you want the ones with feet to last, cut off the feet when the baby grows. If he grows outwards as well as upwards this will not work!

Size ranges vary from shop to shop, but the sizes below serve as a general guide.

Age	Weight	Height
Low birthweight	1.4kg–2.3kg (3–5lb)	—
Newborn	3kg (6.6lb)	Up to 50cm
Up to 1 month	4.5kg (9.9lb)	Up to 56cm
1–3 months	6.5kg (14.3lb)	Up to 62cm
3–6 months	8kg (17.6lb)	Up to 68cm

Boots and Mothercare designs have something for everyone and fit well. We tried these out on a variety of different-shaped babies. An excellent range can also be found in larger branches of Marks & Spencer, Children's World and at Baby Gap.

If your baby's bottom grows quicker than the rest of him, you can buy false bottom extenders to add 3in or 4in (or up to six months) to the use of baby clothes. A pack of four extenders costs £9.95 from the Bright Start catalogue (0171 483 3929).

Packs of three stretchsuits are sold by C&A (terry, £7.99); TESCO, Adams and Mothercare (cotton or terry, £9.99); and Ladybird (Woolworth) at £8.99. Littlewoods offer two in a pack, white or coloured, terry or cotton, for £6.99.

If you don't mind paying a little extra, check out Marks & Spencer's Petit Bébé range.

★★★ Star buy ★★★

Mothercare nightgowns, price £4.99 each, are ideal for either sex. You can change nappies easily without having to undo a mass of poppers each time. They also last longer than stretchsuits. The NCT gowns, £8.50, and the white one could double up as a christening gown.

Scratch Mitts

Only buy these if your newborn is inflicting unsightly damage on himself.

Vests and Bodysuits

Do not buy wrapover vests – the ribbons, though pretty, are fiddly. For tiny babies, Children's World do easy-access wrap-over bodysuits for £3.99.

The best bodysuits are the cotton ones with envelope necks and poppers at the crotch, available at all major outlets. Mothercare sell packs of three, terry or cotton, with short sleeves for £4.99. At C&A you can buy a pack of two in cotton at £2.50.

Cardigans and Jumpers

These are useful for slipping over a stretchsuit on colder days. As they will not be touching the baby's skin, machine-washable wool or a wool–acrylic mixture are the most practical options.

New babies can be very frightened by clothes being pulled over their heads, so look for items that button up the front or have wide openings at the neck and maybe a couple of buttons at the side or back.

Exquisite ribbon fastenings tend to get mangled in the wash and can be difficult to keep done up.

Typical prices for baby knitwear are £8.99 at the Early Learning Centre (100 per cent cotton); £5.99 at Mothercare (100 per cent acrylic) and £5.99 at Boots (72 per cent polyester, 28 per cent cotton).

Outdoor Wear

Babies born in the summer will only need a knitted or padded jacket but winter babies will need a warm snowsuit or a two-piece.

What to look for

- Buy a size larger than you would for other items to allow for extra sweaters.
- Try to find something with feet – baby socks and shoes have a habit of disappearing.
- If you can find a two-piece with trousers that does not have crossover straps, you are lucky indeed. It means you can change a nappy anywhere without having to strip the baby entirely.
- Front zip fastenings are the least fiddly.

Children's World sell a Polar fleece snowsuit (sizes 0–3 months to 18–24 months) at £18.99, and a wadded two-piece set for £15.99.

Footwear

This is not necessary if you have feet on your babygros. If you are buying footwear for warmth, you will find that old-fashioned knitted bootees do not stay on as well as socks, which are definitely the cheapest option. Knee-high socks have a better chance of staying put than short ones.

For serious foot-warming, buy fabric bootees with elasticated ankles. These are often lined with a contrasting fabric or fleece. They are sometimes called padders, after the brand name. Unlined bootees cost from £2.99 and lined ones from £5.

Sock sizes are based on shoe size; generally 00 is newborn and 0–2.5 the next one up. Bootees are sold by age.

Tights

★★★ **Star buy** ★★★

Marks & Spencer cotton-rich (£5.50 for two pairs). They may be more expensive than competing brands, but they are relatively wrinkle-free, they wash well – no bobbles – and their cotton content makes them suitable for every season.

Washing Baby Clothes

The little washtub symbol on the clothes gives the temperature at which you should wash clothes. The line underneath will tell you how vigorously you can wash them.

Washing labels

Line symbol under tub	Strength of wash	Suitable for following fabrics
Line under tub	Medium to gentle wash	For more delicate synthetics and delicate cottons
Broken line under tub	Delicate wash	For wool and silk
No line underneath	Maximum action	Cotton

Washing-Powders and Fabric Conditioners

You may be perfectly happy with your washing-powder and see no reason to change it for washing baby clothes. If you are keen to find something more gentle, look for a product that says on the box something along the lines of 'without enzymes, bleach or brightening agents'. Lux soap flakes (£1.65 for 425g) can be used in the machine and are 99 per cent pure soap. Filetti compact (£1.95 for 500g – equivalent of approximately 870g of normal powder) is a Swiss powder that many swear by. There are also non-biological versions of Persil and Fairy.

If your baby's skin tolerates stronger stuff, specialist pre-wash products such as Bio-tex (£3.29 for 1kg) work well in removing difficult stains before washing.

18 Playtime

Research undertaken for the Carnegie Corporation report, published in 1994, suggests that an infant's brain develops more quickly in the first year than was previously realized. A baby's sensory experiences in her early months literally shape her brain and may have a long-lasting effect on her development.

Animal studies at the University of Illinois show that brains develop differently in more stimulating environments. Young rats which had toys in their cage developed more synapses (connections between brain cells which form the structures that allow you to learn) than rats in empty cages. It works for rats, and it works for brats as well. Toys are not only fun and decorative, they have a crucial role to play in your baby's development.

Stimulating your baby is not about dumping her in a playpen with loads of brightly coloured toys. A newborn is not a blob, but a sponge which absorbs her environment. Spend time with her on your knee, talking to her and showing her pictures. It will all be taken in.

Toys

Give your baby toys that will fascinate her and hold her attention. Here are some general rules to bear in mind.
- Always buy toys made by an established company from a reputable shop. They should bear a BS or CE label showing

that they conform to either British or European standards. Cheap, badly made toys could have easily detachable small parts that pose a threat to your baby.
- Do not give your baby a toy that is too large and sophisticated for her. It may be both frustrating and potentially dangerous when she is too young for it yet bore her by the time she is ready to play with it. The Early Learning Centre clearly marks the suitable age on the wrapping of each toy.
- Playing is about exploring freely. If a toy is so expensive that you are constantly worrying that your baby might break it, don't buy it. Pots, pans, water and old newspapers have given huge amounts of pleasure to generations of infants.

If there is a part of the day or piece of equipment which upsets your baby, you might be able to improve her outlook with a careful choice of toys. If she hates bathtime, buggies or highchairs, some strategically placed toys might persuade her to see them in a new light.

Don't be sexist in your choice of toys, and don't buy anything that you dislike yourself: if it drives you mad in the shop, you will be up the wall by the time it has been home for a few hours. If you do not like it, the chances are that you will not use it with your baby in a positive way, so it will be a waste of money.

Old-Fashioned Toys

If you yearn for well-made wooden toys, telephone for the Hill Toy Company catalogue on 01765 689955 or visit their shop at 71 Abingdon Road, London W8 6AW, tel. 0171 937 8797.

The Baby Basics catalogue offers safe, quality toys for babies and children. Telephone 01703 234949 for a catalogue.

Rocking-horses

Large department stores such as John Lewis and Hamleys sell rocking-horses, or contact the Rocking Horse Shop, Fangfoss, York YO4 5QH, tel. 01759 368737.

Soft Toys

Even if a teddy bear in a local shop looks at you with pleading eyes, don't buy it until you have thought about the following:
- Will it shed hairs?
- Is it washable?
- Are eyes and other parts firmly attached?
- Does it conform to BS5665 and have a CE mark?

It will not be suitable for a baby under one year old if it is made of woollen hair or fibre plush.

Toy Libraries

If you have no idea where to start, contact your local toy library. There are over a thousand in the UK, serving the needs of 110,000 British families. They are ideal for parents who want advice on a variety of developmental toys. Toys can often be borrowed, for a charge of around 20p, until the next session. The additional bonuses of this scheme are that parents meet other families in the area and that children learn to share and play together from an early age.

For details of your nearest toy library, contact the National Association of Toy and Leisure Libraries, 68 Churchway, London NW1 1LT, tel. 0171 387 9592.

Toys for Babies Between One and Three Months

At this age your baby starts to wave his arms and watch his hands and fingers; he kicks vigorously; he may be able to hold up his head a little; he is responsive to familiar voices.

If he wrinkles up his face, looks vacant, turns away, squirms, screams or burps, he may be indicating that he has had enough of a particular toy and you should take it away. Toys with bright lights and loud noises will probably frighten him and make him cry. Look for those that play with light or make gentle sounds or music. He will probably enjoy gentle songs, preferably from you. In addition there are many suitable recordings available.

Mobiles

These can stimulate your baby, encouraging him to watch and reach. Those with soft lullabies might soothe him. Some babies find mobiles disturbing and screech at the sight of them. If yours does this, take the mobile away. Do not buy a mobile if all your baby will be able to see of it is feet. The characters or shapes must be positioned so that the baby can see them properly.

Check that you can attach the mobile as soon as you get it home – not all of them can be fixed to all cot sides. Before you buy it, check that you can take it back if necessary. A mobile which needs batteries is a waste of money. Look for one that is easy to clean. You may want to put it away for another baby after six months.

Mobiles are not intended to be played with, just watched. As soon as your baby can push up and starts to reach out for it, take it down.

★★★ Star buys ★★★

The Infant Stim-Mobile features bold black and white graphics which are reversible and removable, allowing you to build up the complexity of the patterns. It has vertical and horizontal surfaces a baby can see from any angle. Made of plastic and easily washable, it costs £19.99 from Bright Start mail order (0171 483 3929).

The Early Learning Centre's Old Macdonald musical mobile (£14.99) has animals that can be detached for your baby to play with later. Position it over his tummy so that he gets a good view of the animals.

A variation on this is the Tomy Lullaby Light Show (from £16), for use in a darkened room. When you wind it up it plays a tinkling lullabye and the glowing animals are projected on to the walls of the room.

Mirrors

These will be a source of fascination to your baby for months.

★★★ **Star buy** ★★★

The Double Feature mirror by Wimmer Ferguson is probably the largest, safest mirror you can find for use in a cot. You can also use it back to front: on the back it has a seascape of black and white graphics intended to encourage your baby to lift his head. It costs £25 from the Bright Start catalogue (0171 483 3929).

Pictures

Use standard-sized greetings cards you have received as a picture library for the pram. Poke one into the mattress where the baby can see it, and change the picture every few days. Stop this as soon as he can reach out and grasp for objects.

Toys for Babies Between Three and Six Months

By now your baby will be making babbling and cooing noises. She can grasp her feet to play with her toes and sit up when supported. Although she reaches for objects and can hold them briefly, possibly passing them from hand to hand, she may not yet look at them.

★★★ **Star buy** ★★★

The Baby Vision range by Tomy, a series of imaginatively designed toys which a baby can explore unaided, is really worth looking out for. Priced from £2.99 to around £6, they make excellent presents.

Activity Quilts and Mats

Activity mats are brightly patterned mats with detachable toys. Initially they provide a soft, washable surface for your baby to lie on. As she grows, she should become increasingly interested in the toys incorporated in the mat. These usually include a mirror, a squeaky toy and a variety of textured fabrics. Nests are circular mats with an inflated or padded outer ring to support the baby and stop the toys rolling away. These can be bulky to store.

Do not buy one that is too small – anything under 2ft (60cm) square may soon be outgrown. Waterproofing is not essential, but will be useful if you plan to use it outside.

★★★ Star buys ★★★

The Galt Playnest activity ring, price £29.99. For stockists call 0161 4289111.

The Early Learning Centre activity quilt (£14.99) is easily portable, machine-washable and 'full of surprises'.

The Fisher Price Deluxe Discovery quilt (£17 from independent retailers) is smaller but contains a good selection of activities.

Safety

- Do not put mats down in a draughty spot.
- Never carry your baby around in a playmat. Incorporated objects could dig into her.
- Do not use the mat as a blanket. Its synthetic contents could cause the baby to overheat.

Rattles

There are loads of excellent designs available. Good value is the Mothercare telephone. one of a series, which comes in its own clear plastic wallet (£2.99). The Musical Rattle by Tiger Electronics is available from independent retailers. Shaped as a bunny, turtle, elephant or bear, it rolls its eyes and makes music for only £3.99. The Squish is a fascinating rattle, bell, ball and teether that flattens but bounces back into shape. Suitable from birth onwards, it costs £12.50 from the Baby Basics catalogue (01703 234949).

Playsocks

These are animal socks with rattles sewn into the front flaps for your baby to play with. Hypoallergenic and machine-washable, they cost £8.95 a pair from the Bright Start catalogue (0171 483 3929).

Activity Centres

These are boards which incorporate buttons, textures, noises and other activities to entrance a baby. They are usually designed to be fitted on to the side of a cot. Remove it as soon as your baby starts trying to stand up in her cot – as is mentioned elsewhere, she may try to stand on it to get out.

The pre-school activity bear by Matchbox (£13) is particularly popular because it is sturdy, easy to fix, and, most importantly, fun. Your baby will probably not be interested in this type of toy to start with. You will have to show her how it works. If you like everything to match, look out for the Sleepy Bear teether-rattle, the Busy Baby Bear for attaching to your buggy or cot, and the musical Baby Bear.

Tomy's Sunshine activity mobile (£18.99) is extremely good value as it combines a musical mobile with a lively activity centre which can be used either together or separately.

The buggy activity centre is an adjustable bar which clamps on to a pram or buggy and holds a number of bright, robust toys. It costs £9.99 from the Early Learning Centre.

Baby gyms

This frame which suspends and incorporates a number of toys is a hit with most babies. It can be used by a baby in her bouncy chair or lying on her activity mat. Make sure that it is firmly assembled before you allow her to play with it and do not tie extra toys on to it.

The Boots baby gym (£19.99) is probably the most versatile on the market. It is height-adjustable, has a good variety of toys and comes with its own carrier bag.

The Early Learning Centre big activity arch (£17.99) is packed with fun, sensibly positioned toys and is easy to clean.

Fisher Price, Mattel and Tyco all offer popular models.

The Tomy Multi Gym Walker (£29.75) from Argos and toy shops, incorporates six toys in one, including a baby gym, baby walker and activity centre.

Baby Bouncers

These are seats or support units; some you suspend from a door frame or ceiling, others are stand-alone. Baby bouncers allow your baby to jump up and down and exercise her legs. They are pricey, starting at around £19.99, and you are unlikely to be able to use one for more than seven months. Assembly can be fiddly, and some babies hate them.

Others, however, are absolutely ecstatic in their bouncers and for that reason alone the purchase may be worthwhile. If you are seriously considering buying one, it is essential to try before you buy. If you cannot try your baby in a friend's bouncer make sure that the shop will take back one you have bought if she dislikes it.

Stand-alone models can be used inside and outdoors but they take up a lot of room. When fitting a door-hung model, check that the architrave (the moulding surrounding the door frame) will take the weight of a bouncing baby. If the floor slants from one side of the doorway to the other, your baby will only be able to bounce on one leg. If the architraves on either side of the doorway do not match exactly, it might prove difficult to fix on the clamp.

If you are buying a bouncer which hangs from a hook you attach to the ceiling, be careful that you drill into a joist and not plasterboard.

Using a bouncer

- Do not put your baby in the bouncer until she can support her head.
- Your baby should be near enough to the floor for the balls of her feet to rest on it.
- If she wriggles while you are putting her in the bouncer, do not let this distract you from firmly securing her into it.
- If the bouncer is hung in a doorway, make sure that the door cannot swing into your bouncing baby.
- She should not stay in a bouncer for longer than twenty minutes.

★★★ Star buy ★★★

As safety factors depend very much on the conditions in your home, it is not possible to recommend particular brands here. One free-standing model that is widely available is the Tippitoes floor bouncer. This costs around £50 at John Lewis, the Early Learning Centre, Toys R Us and independent nursery shops.

Babywalkers

These are seats with playtrays on a wheeled base which allow babies to move around. They are not suitable for smaller babies.

Playpens

Playpens have largely been superseded by travel cots, soft-sided foldaway cots which can be used for either playing or sleeping in. In particular, look out for the Play Space by Cumfifolda. New on the market, it is produced in the same proportions as a standard playpen and costs around £79.

If you wish to buy a playpen second-hand, look for BS4863.

As the most common accidents with playpens involve children falling as they try to climb out, you need to be sure that:

- The playpen is at least 2ft (60cm) high.
- All bars are intact and not cracked.
- If it has mesh sides, these must be strong and in perfect repair so that fingers cannot be trapped.
- If it has a padded rim, this must be unmarked – babies can choke on bits of fabric or foam.
- Mesh sides must be kept upright so that your baby cannot suffocate in loose fabric.

Never hang toys across the top – strings can strangle. If you put an older baby into the playpen, do not put larger toys inside with him. They might be used as a means of escape.

Bouncy Chairs

These are extremely useful, but only for a short period of time. A bouncy chair holds a baby at a slight angle, enabling him to see the room and any toys you might dangle in front of him.

Because of their short lives, we reckoned that value for money was all-important. The Bettacare bouncing cradle, which includes a head-hugger, is £16.99 from Argos and independent retailers. The Mothercare bouncing cradle is a good size and costs £12.99. You will probably also need a head-hugger. You can buy one in a co-ordinating fabric for £5.99. The Early Learning Centre sells an elegant gingham number that comes with a detachable head-hugger for £19.99 all inclusive.

If you do not want to buy a bouncy chair, you will probably find that a baby car seat performs the same job.

PART TEN
COPING

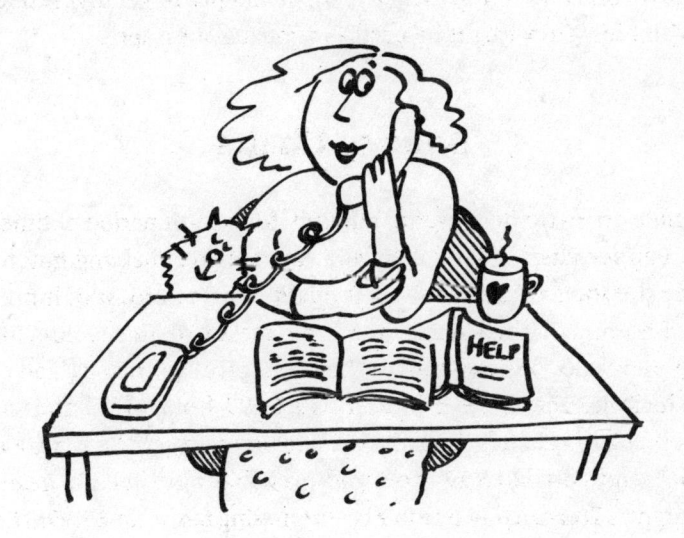

19 Dealing with Problems

The Pressure Pregnancy Places on Relationships

There are men who cannot cope with pregnancy or babies. In some cases, this can lead them to emotionally or physically abuse their partners. If you need to leave the house quickly, you and any children you already have will be welcomed at a local women's refuge. Contact the **Women's Aid Federation**, England, PO Box 391, Bristol BS99 7WS, or one of the following twenty-four-hour telephone numbers:

London: 0171 251 6537.
North of England: 0161 839 8574.
Eire: 01872 3756.
Other Areas: 0117 9633542.
Have a pencil handy to take down further numbers.

Social Services, your local police station, the Samaritans or the Citizens' Advice Bureau should also know of a refuge.

Refuge numbers should never be given out to men.

Losing Your Baby Through Miscarriage or Stillbirth

The threat of miscarriage is the reason why doctors advise you to wait three months before you announce your pregnancy.

According to Tommy's Campaign's statistics, in the UK one in four women suffer miscarriage. Each year, sixty thousand babies are born too soon or too small, and one in a hundred babies is lost through stillbirth.

CARE for Life run a network of centres where women can go for support in the despair that can arise from miscarriages, stillbirths, perinatal deaths or abortion.

Free pregnancy tests are also available. All cases are treated confidentially and no charge is made. Project co-ordinator Camilla Douglas says: 'We are a Christian-based organization, but we are very careful not to impose our views and beliefs on counsellees. We see our role as one coming alongside another at a time of crisis or pain.' Contact them at PO Box 389, Basingstoke, Hampshire RG24 9QF, tel. 01256 850111.

Losing a baby at any stage is a terrible bereavement. Your baby was a real person to you and your family, but other people may forget this, making you feel guilty for grieving.

If you suffer a miscarriage, you can try for another baby as soon as you feel psychologically ready, as long as your doctor confirms that there are no medical reasons to delay.

Fathers often feel unable to express their anguish. They are exhausted from taking on the supporter's role, telling people the news, making necessary arrangements and going to work as if nothing has happened.

Men make up only a small percentage of those calling SANDS (the Stillbirth and Neonatal Death Society) or the Miscarriage Association, although SANDS reports that the number is growing fast. Both of these organizations offer support to both partners, either together or individually.

Such sorrow is often difficult to share, especially when losing a baby can create feelings of guilt in both parents. They fear that they may in some way be responsible but do not want to express this to their partner, for fear of hurting him or her even more.

The excellent booklet *Saying Goodbye to Your Baby*, price £1, and information leaflets and factsheets ranging from *The Loss of your Grandchild* and *Mainly for Fathers* to *Sexual Problems Following a Stillbirth*, are available at a cost of between 10p and 50p from SANDS.

If you need a christening robe to fit a premature baby who has died, contact POPPINS, tel. 0121 778 3482.

Helpful organizations

SANDS (the Stillbirth and Neonatal Death Society), 28 Portland Place, London W1N 4DE, tel. 0171 436 7940, have a helpline open from 9.30 a.m. to 5 p.m. on 0171 436 5881. If you call outside these hours, leave a message on the machine and they will get back to you as soon as they reopen.

The Miscarriage Association keeps lists of local contacts and support groups who can offer help and advice. They are contactable at Clayton Hospital, Wakefield, West Yorkshire WF1 3JS, tel. 01924 200799.

Miscarriage Association of Ireland, 27 Kenilworth Road, Dublin 6, tel. 497 2938.

Compassionate Friends, 53 North Street, Bristol BS3 1EN, tel. 0117 9539639, offer support to parents whose child has died from any cause at any age.

Irish Stillbirth and Neonatal Death Society, Carmichael House, 4 North Brunswick Street, Dublin 7, tel. 837 3367 or 283 1910.

Termination for Abnormality

If you decide to terminate a wanted baby because of foetal abnormality, you are doing it out of love for your baby and your existing family. But this does not make it an easy decision.

SATFA (Support Around Termination For Abnormality) helps parents who discover that their unborn baby is abnormal and can put you in touch with others who have been through a similar experience. Their non-judgemental approach makes their counselling service (tel. 0171 631 0285) a lifeline to many.

You can also contact them for details of their publications and national support network at 73 Charlotte Street, London W1P 1LB, tel. 0171 631 0280.

See above for more organizations that can help.

Cot Death

Cot death or Sudden Infant Death Syndrome (SIDS) is the sudden, unexplained death of an infant. Much has been made of a possible connection between cot mattresses and the incidence of cot death but in tests the Department of Health found no evidence of this. The fall in the number of mortalities is probably due to greater awareness of the possible causes. The Foundation for the Study of Infant Deaths recommends the following:

- Put your baby to sleep on her back.
- Do not smoke during pregnancy or expose your baby to a smoky atmosphere.
- Do not let her get too hot.
- If you think your baby is not well, contact your doctor.
- If you are putting your baby straight into a full-sized cot, make the bed up at the foot of the cot so that she does not have acres of blankets in which to get lost.

Helpful organizations

FSID (Foundation for the Study of Infant Deaths), 14 Halkin Street, London SW1X 7DP. General inquiries: 0171 235 0965; helpline: 0171 235 1721. The FSID funds research into cot death and provides information on relevant issues. The helplines offers advice to parents.

CONI (Care of the Next Infant), Alison Waite, National CONI Organizer, Room C1, Stephenson Unit, Sheffield Children's Hospital, Western Bank, Sheffield S10 2TH. A support organization for parents who have suffered a cot death and now have a new baby.

Irish Sudden Infant Death Society, tel. 874 7007.

Conceiving Again

Help with Problems in Conceiving

A negative pregnancy test does not necessarily mean that there is something wrong or that you will not conceive soon. It is important to remember that the chance of conceiving in any one month for an average 'fertile' couple is only 20 to 25 per cent. An amazing one in every six couples will need advice or medical assistance at some point to help them conceive. Problems with having another baby are also common: up to 15 per cent of couples are unable to have a second child.

Ovulation Tests

To improve chances of becoming pregnant, ISSUE (the National Fertility Awareness Association) suggests:
- Keep fit and healthy and eat a balanced diet.
- If you are overweight, go on a diet.
- If you are underweight, it may be upsetting the function of your ovaries.
- Both prospective parents should cut down on drinking and smoking.

In addition, when planning a pregnancy women should supplement their diet with folic acid. For further advice contact the Foresight Association, an organization concerned with pre-conceptual care.

Easy-to-use ovulation kits can be obtained from your chemist at around £19. These confirm that you are producing eggs and the day of maximum fertility. Refills are available for £11.35.

If you think that a reasonable time has passed and you feel that your doctor is not giving you the treatment that you need, start agitating. According to the National Infertility Awareness campaign, 'To delay referral or progression of patients to the appropriate treatment reduces the likelihood of success. It also wastes NHS resources and valuable time for patients.'

Many health authorities now pay for infertility treatment, but still only an estimated 50 per cent fund IVF, and even then only for a minority of those patients who might benefit from the treatment. If you want to take an active part in campaigning for more infertility treatment to be available on the NHS, contact the National Infertility Awareness Campaign on 0800 716345 for a free information pack. This gives advice on writing to your MP and health authority, plus details of local and national events such as the campaign's annual Focus Week, which in 1996 runs from 16 June.

A 64-page free booklet on fertility problems and ways to resolve them, *So you want to have a baby?*, by obstetrician Roger Neuberg, is available from Serono Laboratories (UK) Ltd, 99 Bridge Road East, Welwyn Garden City, Hertfordshire AL7 1BG, tel. 01707 331972.

A good book to read is *Getting Pregnant*, by Professor Robert Winston, published by Pan at £7.99.

Helpful organizations

ISSUE (the National Fertility Association), 509 Aldridge Road, Great Barr, Birmingham B44 8NA, tel: 0121 344 4414, offers a twenty-four-hour service. **ISSUE** in Dublin: 49 Hermitage Park Road, Lucan, Co. Dublin.

BABIE (the Association for the Betterment of Infertility and Education), PO Box 4TS, London W1A 4TS, helps subfertile couples with any difficulties. They provide counselling, a free helpline, factsheets and medical facilities.

CHILD (Charity for Infertility, Education and Counselling), Charter House, 43 St Leonards Road, Bexhill-on-Sea, East Sussex TN40 1JA, tel. 01424 732361. A twenty-four-hour answering service offers information, advice and support, and produces a series of factsheets on infertility subjects.

Foresight, the association for the promotion of preconceptual care, 28 The Paddock, Godalming, Surrey GU7 1XD, tel. 01483 427839.

Women with general health queries, including abnormal smear tests, reproduction problems, osteoporosis, sterilization questions etc., should contact **Women's Health**, an inquiry service supplying information on a wide range of topics. Women's Health is committed to assisting in a supportive manner, helping women to make informed decisions about their health. You can either write for information, enclosing a large SAE, to Women's Health, 52 Featherstone Street, London EC1, or telephone them on 0171 251 6580. All inquiries are answered by women. Their reference library can be visited by appointment.

Pregnancy tests

Home Pregnancy Tests

If you use a home pregnancy test, be sure to follow it up with a test at your doctor's. It is not uncommon for a test to be negative when you are in fact pregnant. Positive test results tend to be more reliable.

Products on the market include Clearblue, Boots Own, One Step and First Response. They cost between £8.45 and £10.95.

PLUS POINTS
* Ninety-nine per cent accurate.
* Quick and simple.
* They can be used at any time of the day.
* They can be used as early as the first day of a missed period.
* Completely private.

MINUS POINTS
* Expensive.
* If they give a false negative result you may not know that you're pregnant for quite a while.

Other Options

- **LIFE** (Save the Unborn Child) offer free pregnancy testing. This organization also provides counselling to help pregnant women resist the pressure to have an abortion and a post-abortion counselling service. Their head office is Life House, Newbold Terrace, Leamington Spa, Warwickshire CV32 4EA, tel. 01926 421587/311667/316737. They also have a national helpline, open from 9 a.m. to 9 p.m., on 01926 311511.

- **Brook Advisory Centres** offer young people under twenty-five free pregnancy tests and confidential counselling. If no centre is listed in your telephone directory, their head office will tell you about the best alternative in your area. Their head office is at 165 Gray's Inn Road, London WC1X 8UD, tel. 0171 833 8488. Their helpline is on 0171 713 9000.

- Your own GP can provide a free serum or blood pregnancy test. This is the most accurate test available – almost 100 per cent accuracy as early as one week after conception is claimed. A doctor might also give you a medical examination to confirm the test findings.

- **Family Planning Clinics** give free pregnancy tests, but they may only do so if you have already been attending the clinic for contraception. You can get a full list of clinics from the Family Planning Association, 27–35 Mortimer Street, London W1N 7RJ, tel. 0171 636 7866.

- The **Pregnancy Advisory Service**, 11–13 Charlotte Street, London W1P 1HD, tel. 0171 637 8962, charge £7 for a pregnancy test.

- The **British Pregnancy Advisory Service** charge £8 for a pregnancy test. Their head office is at Austy Manor, Wooton, Wawen, Solihull, West Midlands B95 6BX, tel. 01564 793225.

- **CURA Pregnancy Counselling** (Eire), tel. 671 0598.

- Chemists often offer pregnancy testing. If it is not advertised in the window, ask the counter staff. At around £5 to £6, it is often cheaper than buying a home kit – you can usually get the result within an hour. Boots do not generally have a pregnancy-testing service.

> !!! If your periods have stopped and you are experiencing pain, be sure to check with your doctor that you do not have an ectopic pregnancy. This is when the foetus starts to develop outside the womb. Symptoms include cramps, vaginal bleeding, feelings of nausea and dizziness. Some women also experience shoulder pains and feelings of rectal pressure.

Adoption and Fostering

If you are unable to have a baby at all, you might like to consider the following options.

Fostering

Being a foster carer involves looking after a child in your own home for a short period of time. You work with the child's parents and the fostering agency to provide the best environment for the child. You are given an allowance by the local authority, but payment varies depending on where you live.

Adopting

Adopting a child means that you become his legal parents. He has the same rights and entitlements as any member of your family. You have as much responsibility as if he were your own flesh and blood.

There are only a few healthy babies in England and Wales available for adoption. In 1992, 7,342 children were adopted but only around 661 of them were under one year old, and in Scotland, of a total of 786 children, only 63 were under a year. Even if you have set your heart on adopting a baby you may be unsuccessful. If you want to adopt a child with special needs, BAAF (British Agencies for Adoption and Fostering) publish a bimonthly newspaper called *Be My Parent*, which lists details of children in need of a home. Parent to Parent, the national self-help and information organization (see below), also publishes a monthly magazine for potential parents.

There are no adoption agencies in Britain that will help you arrange to adopt a baby from overseas, but the Home Office provide a special leaflet, RON117, about adopting from abroad.

Helpful organizations

British Agencies for Adoption and Fostering, Skyline House, 200 Union Street, London SE1 0LX, tel. 0171 593 2000.

BAAF Scottish Centre, 40 Shandwick Place, Edinburgh EH2 4RT, tel. 0131 225 9285.

Parent to Parent, Information on Adoption Services, Lower Boddington, Daventry, Northamptonshire NN11 6YB, tel. 01327 260295.

National Foster Care Association, Leonard House, 5–7 Marshalsea Road, London SE1 1EP, tel. 0171 828 6266.

Home Office Immigration and Nationality Department, Lunar House, Wellesley Road, Croydon, Surrey CR9 2BY, tel. 0181 686 0688.

The **Catholic Children's Society**, 49 Russell Hill Road, Purley, Surrey CR8 2XB, tel. 0181 668 2181. Some mothers request that their children are placed with Catholic families.

When Things Go Wrong with the Birth

In a small percentage of cases, births do go wrong, and the baby may die or suffer brain damage as a result.

If you have concerns about the service you are receiving, first tell the people involved – your doctor or postnatal clinic. If that does not work, contact the general manager or chief executive of the Family Health Services Authority or hospital.

The Health Information Service on 0800 665544 will explain how you can complain.

Your local community health council can also provide help and advice. Their contact details will be listed under Community Health Council in your local telephone directory.

The Birth Crisis Line is for people who feel that they have been disempowered or mutilated by a traumatic birth experience. Tel. 01865 300266.

Suing the Hospital

Unfortunately there are occasions when the delivery of a baby is mismanaged, resulting in injuries to the baby or the mother, or both. When this happens the new mother may wish to make a claim against the hospital for damages. If there is a serious injury it might be essential for her to claim, because she may need financial assistance to pay for specialist nursing care and other expenses arising from the injuries.

If you think that you have a claim, or would like to find out if you do, it is worth seeking a preliminary discussion with a solicitor who specializes in this area of law. Your local Citizens' Advice Bureau will probably have a list of them. The solicitor should be able to give you an initial assessment of your chances of success and answer any queries that you may have. Many solicitors, irrespective of the question of Legal Aid or funding the claim, run a scheme whereby they will give you a free initial half-hour for a discussion.

Questions to ask
- Will my claim be successful?
- What can I claim for?

- How long will the claim take?
- How much will it cost?

Will my claim be successful?

All claims for damages for personal injuries are based on the law of negligence. The test of whether someone has been negligent is essentially whether they have failed to do something which they ought to have done, or have done something they ought not to have done. If injury has apparently been caused by someone involved in the delivery failing to do something or doing something wrong, the likelihood is that there is a justifiable claim to be made.

What can I claim for?

Damages are made up of two parts: the first is for the actual pain, injury, suffering and loss of amenity caused to mother or baby; the second for financial expenditure.

The amount of the damages for the injury is based on medical reports which will be obtained to show its nature and extent and for how long it is likely to continue. The other part of the claim – for expenditure created by the injury – very often represents the greater sum.

In very serious cases, the claim will include the purchase of special accommodation, for example, a bungalow where it is apparent that the injury prevents the victim from using stairs; a specially adapted car for someone who is unable to sit properly or who needs to sit in a wheelchair; the wheelchair itself; the cost of nursing care, sometimes on a twenty-four-hour basis; the costs of medication, and all other expenses which have come about because of the injury. These may also include loss of earnings for the mother or anyone else who has to take time off work or give up his or her job to look after either the mother or the baby.

Even if a mother has not herself suffered physical injury during the delivery, she may be able to show that she has suffered emotional trauma because of the injury to her baby. If so, she may have a claim in respect of emotional trauma.

How long will it take?

Obviously, the sooner a claim is started, the sooner it is likely to be concluded. Immediately after the delivery, it may be difficult for the new mother to come to terms with the fact that something has gone seriously wrong and thus difficult to take the first steps towards making a claim.

The more detailed the mother's recollection of events, and the father's, assuming he was present at the delivery, the easier the job of bringing a claim will be. It is therefore a good idea to write down as soon as possible a full account of what happened while it is still fresh in your memory. The hospital will have notes and records, which will include very specific information such as the print-out for the foetal heart rate, the times when checks were made on mother and baby, what drugs were given and when, etc., but the human side, from the mother's point of view, is still very important.

The advantage of getting things moving as soon as possible cannot be overstated. There are time limits for bringing claims. The court proceedings must be started within three years of the date of the injury, or of when it first became apparent that injury had occurred (for example, if something is revealed by a postnatal medical check-up). This three-year rule does not apply to anyone under the age of eighteen, so children have three years from their eighteenth birthday to bring a claim themselves, but in normal circumstances matters should not be left that long. The rule also does not apply to anyone who needs permanent care because of mental incapacity. Therefore time never runs out for someone who suffered serious permanent brain damage at birth, but it is best to get on with the claim as soon as possible nonetheless.

The usual assumption is that these cases take a long time because the law is a slow and cumbersome process and lawyers are not the quickest of individuals when it comes to processing claims. Whatever the truth of this, the claim cannot in any case be concluded until it is possible to establish how the long-term future of the mother or baby has been affected. If a baby is born with serious injuries, this may be impossible to predict before it achieves infancy, or perhaps even pre-adolescence. Therefore it is not safe to finally settle the claim until it is known how long the damages need to last and exactly what has to be claimed for.

However, it is not usually necessary to wait until the very end of the process before any damages can be obtained. If the hospital is prepared to admit that it was to blame, which is not as uncommon as might be thought, or if it is not prepared to admit culpability, but the lawyers are able to have the question of blame decided by the court before the final valuation is possible, and the court finds for the claimant, application can be made for payment on account of the final damages figure.

How much will it cost?

The question of financing claims of this sort is inevitably a difficult one, because court proceedings are expensive, and particularly so in such cases. Not only do the solicitors' fees have to be found at an early stage, a barrister is also likely to become involved. In addition it may be necessary to obtain reports from various medical experts to prove the mismanagement of the birth and the mother's and baby's condition, and to give an assessment of what will be required for the future.

Traditionally, Legal Aid has been available to fund such claims, and this will be applied for by a solicitor on the mother's behalf. Entitlement to Legal Aid is decided by two factors:

- **Whether there is a good claim.** It is not always obvious at the first meeting with the solicitor that there is a cast-iron claim, but the solicitor making the application for Legal Aid needs to be able to advise the Legal Aid Board that he considers there is a good chance of success, and will do so from what the mother is able to tell him.

- **Finance.** If the mother is the injured party, her income and capital are taken into consideration. It is worth inquiring about eligibility for Legal Aid, but as a very general rule, anybody who has a joint income with her spouse, if applicable, of more than about £8,000 a year may not qualify.

The position is different for the baby. While the application has to be made on his behalf, he has an entitlement to Legal Aid in his own right, and therefore, assuming he has a good case, he is unlikely to be denied Legal Aid for financial reasons, as very few babies have an income or any capital of their own.

It is not advisable to make a claim through the courts if Legal Aid is not available, because generally the party who loses not only has to pay his or her own lawyers and expert costs, but also the other side's. The loser therefore has two lots of fees to find, and no damages from which to meet them.

A new arrangement known as conditional fees may be available. This is an agreement with the solicitor that if the claim is not successful he will not charge for his services. It involves taking out an insurance policy to cover the other side's fees. This type of funding is an alternative worth discussing with a solicitor.

This section was contributed by Fred Isherwood, an associate with Edge & Ellison, one of Britain's leading firms of solicitors. One of their areas of expertise is personal injury and negligence claims. They can be contacted at Regent Court, Regent Street, Leicester LE1 7BR, tel. 0116 247 0123. Please note that the law may differ in Scotland, Northern Ireland and Eire.

Helpful organizations

Birth Defects Foundation, Chelsea House, Westgate, London W5 1DR, tel. 0181 862 0198.

Contact a Family, 170 Tottenham Court Road, London W1P 0HA, tel. 0171 383 3555. This group will put you in touch with local and national support networks and link you with families with similarly affected children, especially those with very rare syndromes. They offer general information on special needs and are glad to act as a sounding-board.

Cerebral Palsy Helpline: 0800 626216.

Child Death Helpline: freephone 0800 282 986. The helpline is open every evening from 7 p.m. to 10 p.m. and on Wednesdays 10 a.m. to 1 p.m.

'Baby Blues' and Postnatal Depression

After having a baby, about 50 per cent of all mothers experience a depression that can last from a few hours to a few days. This is often known as the 'Blues'. If it lasts any longer, you *must* see a doctor – you may be suffering from postnatal depression. This is a serious illness, but it can be successfully treated.

Baby Blues

The blues are thought to be caused by a combination of hormonal change, exhaustion and contrasting extreme emotions – apprehension, great joy and anxiety. You feel tearful and tired, but symptoms disappear after a few hours or days.

Help yourself by having a rest during the day. If the baby goes to sleep, be sure that you do too. Have hot, sweet drinks at regular intervals, and do not forget to eat. Go for a short walk every day. Gentle exercise can help. Do not wait until you feel desperate to ask you health visitor or doctor for advice.

Postnatal Depression

This can strike at any time up to a year after the birth. Sufferers feel unable to cope with domestic demands, frequently burst into tears and experience panic attacks. Simple tasks seem a struggle. You may lose interest in sex, your partner or your baby. It can last for over a year, but even without treatment it will pass. Partners may be too exhausted themselves to realize that the new mother is suffering.

The Defeat Depression Campaign has launched a leaflet called *Postnatal Depression*, which explains symptoms, causes and treatment. Send an SAE to Mrs Mary Ayres, The Royal College of Psychiatrists, 17 Belgrave Square, London SW1X 8PG.

Helpful organizations

The Association for Postnatal Illness, 25 Jerdan Place, London SW6 1BE, tel. 0171 386 0868.

Postnatal Distress Association of Ireland, Carmichael House, 4 North Brunswick Street, Dublin 7, tel. 872 7172.

MAMA (Meet-A-Mum Association), 14 Willis Road, Croydon, Surrey CRD 2XX, tel. 0181 665 0357 (9.30 a.m. to 1 p.m.).

PMS Help, PO Box 160, St Albans, Hertfordshire AL1 4UQ. For women who suffer from premenstrual syndrome and postnatal depression.

Eating Your Placenta to Ward Off Postnatal Depression

Most mammals eat their placentas, as do various tribes in developing countries. In Britain it is viewed by some as a way to counteract the devastating effects of severe postnatal depression. The theory is that, just as hormone-replacement therapy works to assist women through the menopause, eating the placenta immediately replaces the natural progesterone that you lose giving birth.

Women who suffered from postnatal depression and psychosis after having their first child and ate their placenta over a five-day period after the birth of a second, report a marked improvement in their general physical wellbeing.

Dr Walter Barker of the Early Childhood Development Unit at Bristol University says there are strong reasons to suggest that eating some or all of the placenta may be very healthy. 'A mother has the right to ask that her placenta be washed in cold water, wrapped in a clean plastic bag and returned to her to take home. It is essential that her own placenta is returned.' He believes there is a possibility that postnatal depression is caused by the new mother's deficiency of zinc and vitamins – a woman's zinc level drops particularly strongly two or three days before the birth as more zinc is transferred to the baby. As an alternative for those who cannot bear the thought of eating their placenta, Dr Barker suggests taking mineral and vitamin supplements, especially zinc, during the weeks following the birth. If you have smoked heavily during pregnancy, the placenta may also contain a sizeable amount of the poisonous mineral cadmium. You may be advised by your doctor or midwife not to eat it.

If you want to try eating your placenta, here are some serving suggestions from Dr Barker.

Raw placenta

Some mothers like to eat pieces of placenta raw, especially on the first day or two after birth, and then to start cooking the rest.

Cut pieces of raw placenta into cubes or strips and serve with cucumber, carrot slices or other salads. You can also dip pieces of it into a tasty oil or thick sauce, such as an avocado or salad sauce, to add flavour.

Cooked placenta

To fry, treat placenta much as you would liver, cutting it into strips and frying it lightly. To add flavour cook it with onions and gravy, or cut it into strips and fry it lightly in oil with a little garlic and wine, add cream and serve it with rice (preferably brown).

You can also cut it into cubes or strips and make it into a *mild* curry with a few vegetables. Serve it with brown rice. Strong curries or spices can cause problems for a breastfed baby.

Placenta can be served cooked or raw with red kidney, haricot or other beans for a tasty meal. Add a pasta for energy balance.

Remember
- Wrap and store the placenta in the fridge.

Sleep Problems

If your baby won't sleep, a sleep clinic may be able to help. These are free and are run by specially trained health visitors. Your own health visitor should be able to tell you if there is a clinic in your area – there may be one attached to your local hospital. Otherwise write to the Karvol Sleep Management Service, Keene Communications, 37 Golden Square, London W1R 4AH. The service holds a national register of sleep clinics.

A useful book is *Solve Your Child's Sleep Problems* by Dr Richard Ferber (Dorling Kindersley, £6.99).

The Baby Sleep Tight cassette plays womb music and can be used to settle a baby. It costs £6.99 from Sound Ideas mail order, tel. 01703 333405; Sound Ideas will do their best to post it to you within twenty-four hours of receiving the order. Otherwise, make a cassette of 'white noise' such as vacuuming – this is very easy if you have a double cassette machine. You simply tape yourself cleaning on one tape and then record it repeatedly on the other.

The sound of children playing might also fascinate and calm your baby.

Cranial osteopathy works for some sleepless babies. See pages 124–5.

Another option is to buy a swinging chair such as the Advantage Swing, £99.99, or the Cumfi Swing 90, which doubles as a car seat.

Helpful organizations

The **Cry-sis** helpline is manned between 6 p.m. and 11 p.m., on 0171 404 5011. Their publications department (01322 401987) supply a number of publications including a crying baby checklist that contains hints to settle your baby.

Colic

About 20 per cent of babies get colic, drawing their legs up to their tummies as they scream with pain. There are no guaranteed methods to alleviate the symptoms; however, the following may help.

- **Cooled, boiled water.** Give this either in a bottle or on a teaspoon.
- **Disposable bottle systems.** As the baby sucks the milk out of the bag it collapses, ensuring that he does not take in air with his feed. Sucking in air is thought to cause colic, although there is still no medical proof that this is the case.
- **Medications and drinks.** Try Infacol and other branded gripe waters, mint tea made with boiled, warm water or Chamomilia herbal drops (see Chapter 11).

Cranial massage can also work wonders (see Complementary Medicines and Therapies in Chapter 6).

APPENDICES

Pregnancy Checklist

For full details, consult the appropriate sections in the main text.

Months 1–3

Health checks

- Take a pregnancy test if your period has not occurred.
- Take folic acid tablets if you are not doing so already.
- Watch your diet.
- Stop drinking, smoking and taking recreational drugs.
- At the end of month 3, you may be offered an ultrasound scan or CVS (chorionic vilus sampling).

Your job and benefits

- Find out if you qualify for statutory maternity pay, maternity allowance or incapacity benefit. Your benefits agency will probably be unable to give on-the-spot advice but will post you their findings.
- If you work with dangerous substances which could harm your unborn child, consider telling your employer of your pregnancy so that he or she can try to find you an alternative – equivalent – job.

Your baby

By the end of month 3, your baby's systems are well developed. She is around 7.5cm long and weighs around 18g.

Don't forget

- If you need dental treatment you must tell your dentist that you are pregnant. You should be seen without charge.
- Apply for free prescriptions from your GP (you will need form FW8, available from your health visitor, doctor or midwife).
- If you are already on income support, find out if you qualify for additional benefits.

Months 4–6

Health checks

You should be offered:
- An AFP (alpha foetoprotein) test.
- A full foetal scan to check in detail the anatomy of your baby.
- The triple test or the triple test plus. This may be followed by an amniocentesis.
- You will probably have a scan at this point.

Your job and benefits

- Fourteen weeks before your baby is due, ask your GP or midwife for form MAT B1 (maternity certificate). This shows when your baby is due. If you are employed, give it to your employer to protect your statutory maternity pay. NB: weeks are calculated as seven twenty-four-hour periods starting at midnight on the Saturday before your baby is due.
- If you are not eligible for SMP, now is the time to apply for maternity allowance. You will need form MA1, available from your maternity or child-health clinic or benefits agency.

Your baby

By the end of month 6 your baby is 33cm long and weighs just over half a kilo. His growth has slowed down, but he begins to mature. He has well-developed arms and legs.

Don't forget

Month 4:
- Book your antenatal class now to be sure of a place.
- Ring for maternity-wear catalogues.
- If you want to learn about parenting, contact PIPPIN to see if there is a course in your area.

Month 5:
- If you want a particular pram or cot and it is made overseas (e.g., Mamas & Papas or Bébé Confort), order it now for collection later.

Months 7–9

Health checks

- You will probably have more frequent health checks.
- If you have not been shown pelvic floor exercises, ask your midwife for instructions. Train yourself to do them at regular intervals (for example, if you are driving, at every red traffic light).

Your job and benefits

You can start maternity leave eleven weeks before the birth (i.e., in the twenty-ninth week of pregnancy).

Your baby

By month 8, your baby will have fat under her skin. She may have hair on her head and nails that need cutting. An average baby is about 50cm long and weighs around 3.4kg at delivery.

Don't forget

- Pack your bags and list emergency telephone numbers.

- Organize your home. Prepare a spare bed if someone is coming to help out, put food in the freezer and vases at the ready.
- You may want to find out about ordering a TENS machine. Boots have a rental service.
- Buy a bath safety mat. It will help you if you are worried about slipping as you get in and out of the bath and it will be useful for your baby later on.
- Join a good video club – you will be very dependent on home entertainment.
- Find out if any of your local shops deliver.
- Organize childcare if you are returning to work.

After the Birth

Remember

- Register the baby's birth.
- Be sure to claim all benefits to which you are entitled before it becomes too late.
- At least seven weeks after your estimated due date, write to your employer stating that you will be coming back to work. This protects your right to return.

The Essentials

What you should consider buying before your baby arrives:

Baby Clothes

6 to 8 stretchsuits or gowns
6 vests (or bodysuits with poppers at the crotch)
2 cardigans in knitted acrylic
4 pairs of socks
3 bibs

Summer babies
A lightly padded jacket
1 sun hat

Winter babies
1 two-piece or all-in-one snowsuit
1 hat-and-mitten set

Bathtime
1 towelling 'cuddlerobe'
Cotton-wool pads

Cotton buds
Baby scissors/clippers

Bedding
A cot
3 cotton cellular blankets

4 fitted bottom sheets
4 top sheets

Bottle Feeding
Teats
6 bottles
Bottle brush

Sterilizer unit
Formula milk

Breastfeeding
Nursing bras
Breast pads

2 feeding bottles and teats

Changing Equipment
Changing mat
Nappies
Nappy-rash cream

Bucket or bin for used nappies, or nappy sacks

Medicine chest
A thermometer
Baby paracetamol/Calpol

First-aid kit

Travel
A pram or buggy for newborn use

A car seat or baby carrier

Good Buys For Parents of Multiples

A large changing bag.

A large travelcot or playpen. If the phone goes or the doorbell rings, you must have somewhere safe to put them.

A bouncy chair. You can bounce one baby in the chair using your foot while feeding the other.

Dimmer switch in the bedroom. You do not want to wake up one baby during the night while you are feeding the other.

Safety items around the house. You may be able to watch one baby the whole time, but not more. Treat the kitchen like a war zone.

Baby car seats. Buy the lightest baby carriers with rigid handles. Carry them in the crook of your arm. Elasticated handles will be harder to manage.

Moses baskets. Carrycots are too heavy and expensive. If you need to carry your babies round your home while they sleep during the day, or want them by your bed at night, go for Moses baskets – the largest palm baskets (and stands) you can find. Wicker ones are bigger than the palm variety, but tend to be considerably dearer and heavier.

Cotbeds. These are better than cots as they will save hassle when it is time to transfer the babies to something larger. They also allow each baby to go at his or her own pace. Choose a cotbed with adjustable mattress heights so that you are not always bending down into the cotbeds.

Changing tables. Especially if you have had a Caesarean, you must ensure that you can change your babies at waist level. However, remember to observe the safety advice on pages 213–14.

Further Reading

We asked Waterstone's, dedicated to excellence in bookselling from their shops located in nearly every major town in Britain and Ireland, for their views. A combination of staff recommendation (there are lots of parents at Waterstone's) and popularity with customers produced the following list of 'musts' for all parents, carers and parents-to-be.

Baby and Child by Penelope Leach (Penguin, £13). Penelope Leach has written a range of very sensible publications and it is worth particularly recommending this book on grounds of popularity alone.

The Baby Book of Ireland is a comprehensive and practical guide for mothers in Ireland (Madison Books, £8.99).

The Complete Baby and Toddler Meal Planner by Annabel Karmel (Ebury Press, £9.99). The title is self-explanatory and the contents worthwhile. Highly regarded in many busy homes.

Dorling Kindersley Complete Mother and Baby Care (Dorling Kindersley, £14.99) makes a particularly good gift for the mother-to-be, offering up-to-date guidance in an attractive and straightforward style. Lots of photographs and illustrations support the text, in classic Dorling Kindersley style. The publisher is well known for its high standards in information books, and this one is no exception.

The Great Ormond Street Book of Baby and Childcare (Bodley Head, £13.99) covers every ailment, developmental phase and potential practical problem in child-rearing. Sensible and no-nonsense, it boasts the medical expertise to give real confidence to anxious adults.

The New Baby Care Book by Miriam Stoppard (Dorling Kindersley, £7.99). Miriam Stoppard is an acknowledged expert on pregnancy and babycare, and has a string of successful books to her name. This comprehensive and affordable title is one of the most popular with Waterstone's customers.

Pregnancy by Gordon Bourne (Pan, £8.99) is a comprehensive guide to pregnancy. As it is written by an obstetrician, it tends to be more detailed in its analysis of medical aspects.

Solve Your Child's Sleep Problems by Richard Ferber (Dorling Kindersley, £6.99) offers practical solutions for frazzled carers, including long-term action plans for the really determined infant insomniac. There are quite a few books on this subject, but Ferber seems to offer really winning suggestions, and meaningful comfort for the insoluble problems.

Toddler Taming by Dr Christopher Green (Arrow, £8.99). Waterstone's sells more copies of this book than of any other childcare title. It is an absolutely indispensable battlefield guide to surviving a child's less likeable habits and phases. Dr Green is calm, very funny and doesn't assume the patience of a saint in his readers, but campaigns for good and loving parenting in regular human beings.

All of the above titles are also available from Waterstone's mail order on 01225 448595, which will supply any book in print anywhere in the world.

Magazines for Mothers and their Babies

All magazines are a good source of interesting articles, helpful hints, useful tips, special offers and free gifts. These are priced between £1.35 and £2.50. Monthly titles include: *Our Baby*, *Parents*, *Practical Parenting*, *First Steps*, *Mother & Baby*.

Other baby magazines which are just as good but appear less frequently are: *Your Complete Guide to Pregnancy & Birth*, *The She Magazine Guide to Having a Baby*, *The NCT's Pregnancy Plus*, *Baby Magazine*.

Index

abortion, 319, 324
accessories, prams and buggies, 285–7
accidents, 105–13
Active Birth Movement, 41–2
activity centres, 311
activity quilts and mats, 309–10
acupuncture, 121
adoption, 325–6
aerials, 231–2
AFP (alpha foetoprotein) test, 34
AIMS (Association for Improvements in the Maternity Services), 18, 21
air travel, 66, 294–5
alcohol, 51
Alexander Technique, 121–2
all-terrain buggies, 280–1
allergies, 255
amniocentesis, 35–6
anaesthetics, 143–5
anencephaly, 34
animals, 114–16
antenatal care: disabled women, 45
  National Health Service, 20–7
  private medicine, 28–30
  tests and screening, 30–7
  and work, 68
antenatal classes, 38–42, 166
  disabled women, 45–6
antibiotics, 53
antidepressants, 54
aquanatal classes, 42
aromatherapy, 122–3
ASDA, 89–90
Association for Postnatal Illness, 333

asthma, 53
au pairs, 181–2

BAAF Scottish Centre, 326
BABIE, 322
'baby blues', 332
baby bouncers, 312–13
baby-carriers, 265–6
baby diners, 260–1
baby foods, 253–7
baby gyms, 311–12
baby monitors, 230–2
Baby Products Association, 104
baby seats, 270–3
baby wipes, 193
babygros, 300–1
babysitting, 181
babywalkers, 313
Bach flower remedies, 124
backache, 58
banks, 81–2
Bart's Test, 34–5
bathrooms, safety, 111
baths:
  accessories, 161
  baby baths, 199–200
  toiletries, 55–6
  thermometers, 200
beauty care, 54–8
bedding: cots, 225, 340
  prams and buggies, 286–7
bedrooms, safety, 111–12
beds, cotbeds, 220–1, 341
benefits, 72–6, 168
BhS, 90
bibs, 160–1, 252

bicycling, 287–90
birth *see* labour
Birth Crisis Line, 327
Birth Defects Foundation, 331
birth plans, 137–8
blankets, 225
bleeps, hiring, 101–2
BLISS, 149–50
blood tests, 32, 34
bodysuits, 301
books, 161, 342–3
booster seats, 260
bootees, 303
Boots, 90–1
borrowing money, 81
bottle feeding, 243–53, 341
bottle-warmers, 249–50
bouncers, 312–13
bouncy chairs, 314
brain, development, 305
bras, 58–61
breastfeeding, 149, 235–43, 341
breasts: bras, 59–62
　breast pads, 238–9
　breast pumps, 240–2
　breast shells, 239
breathing techniques, 139
British Acupuncture Council, 121
British Agencies for Adoption and Fostering, 326
British Institute of Learning Disabilities (BILD), 46
British Pregnancy Advisory Service, 324
British Standard Institute, 102–4
Brook Advisory Centres, 324
brown patches, skin (chloasma), 56
bubble bath, 201
buggies, 279–87, 292
buggy liners, 286
building societies, 77–8
bumpers, 226

cabbage leaves, engorged breasts, 240
Caesarean, 21, 138, 144, 145
Caesarean Support Group, 21
caffeine, 51
carbon-monoxide detectors, 109

CARE for Life, 318
carriage prams, 276–7
carriers, 265–6
carrycots:
　covers, 286
　restraints, 270
cars, 295–6
　seatbelt guides, 67
　car seats, 266–73, 295–6
cat nets, 286
Catholic Children's Society, 326
cats, 115–16
Centre for Pregnancy Nutrition, 48, 53
Cerebral Palsy Helpline, 332
ceremonies to mark the birth, 155–9
chairs: bouncy chairs, 314
　highchairs, 258–62
　nursing chairs, 213
changing bags, 195–6
changing tables, 342
changing units, 213–14
cheese, 49–50
chemical sterilizers, 250
CHILD, 322
child benefit, 75
Child Death Helpline, 332
childcare, 169–84
childminders, 169–72
Children's World, 91–2
chiropractic, 124
chloasma, 56
Choices in Childcare, 183–4
chorionic villus sampling (CVS), 36
christenings, 155–6
Citizen's Charter, 17–18
clothes: baby, 130, 160, 299–304, 340–1
　for breastfeeding, 237–8
　maternity clothes, 62–5
　premature babies, 149
　washing, 303–4
coach travel, 296
coconut-hair mattresses, 224
coir mattresses, 224
colds, 53, 204
colic, 336
comforters, 228–9

Community Health Council, 18
Compassionate Friends, 319
complementary medicine, 120–7, 143
conception problems, 321–3
CONI (Care of the Next Infant), 320
consultants, 21, 29
Consumer Safety Unit, 113
Contact a Family, 331–2
contracts: childcare, 171–2
    nannies, 177–8, 179–80
convertible prams, 277
cordocentesis, 36–7
cosmetics, 55–8
cosytoes, 286
cot death, 221, 320
cotbeds, 221–2
cots, 111–12, 218–21
    bumpers, 226
    mattresses, 221–4, 320
    travel cots, 292–3, 313
cotton buds, 201
cotton wool, 201
coughs, 53
counselling, genetic, 37–8
cow's milk, 257
cradle cap, 204
cranial osteopathy, 124–5
creches, 181
credit cards, 81
crockery, 160
Cry-sis, 336
Cuidiu/Irish Childbirth Trust, 41
CURA Pregnancy Counselling (Eire), 324
curtains, nurseries, 210–11
cycling, 287–90
cystitis, 55

dairy products, 48, 49, 50
Daycare Trust, 183
death: cot death, 320
    miscarriage and stillbirth, 317–19
Debenhams, 92
decorating nurseries, 207–13
dental treatment, 75–6, 202
depression, postnatal, 332–5
diabetes, 54
diet see food

disabled women, 45–7
dismissal from work, 71
disposable bottle feeding systems, 247–8
disposable nappies, 128, 187–9
doctors: consultants, 21, 29
    GPs, 19–22
dogs, 114, 116
Domino scheme, 22
doors, safety, 106–7
Double Test, 34–5
Down's syndrome, 33, 35, 36
drawing rooms, safety, 112–13
drinks, caffeine, 51
drugs: during birth, 139, 144
    free prescriptions, 75–6
    during pregnancy, 52–3
dummies, 228–9

Early Learning Centre, 93
ectopic pregnancy, 325
eggs, safety, 50
electricity, safety, 113
empathy belly, 164–5
employment, 68–71
entonox, 143
environment, 117–20, 128–34
epidural anaesthetic, 144
epilepsy, 54
episiotomy, 138, 150
equipment: baby food, 256, 258
    British standards, 102–4
    environmentally friendly, 131–2
    hiring, 100–2
    holidays, 291–4, 295
Equipped, 47
equity-based investments, 81–5
essential oils, 122–3
European standards, 103–4
expressing milk, 240–3
extended maternity absence, 70

fabric conditioners, 304
fabrics, decorating nurseries, 210–11
family planning clinics, 324
fatherhood, 164–7, 317
Federation of Services for Unmarried Parents and Children, 169

feet: babies' footwear, 303
  care of, 58
  reflexology, 127
ferries, 296
fertility problems, 321–5
fibre mattresses, 223
finances: benefits, 72–6
  financial planning, 76–86
  multiple pregnancies, 43–4
fire: extinguishers, 110
  smoke detectors, 108–9
first aid, 105–6
first-aid kit, 203, 342
fish, 51
fleeces, 226
floors: nurseries, 212–13
  safety, 107
flowers, 158
foam mattresses, 222
foam wedges, 226
foetal alcohol syndrome, 51
folic acid, 48–9, 321
food: allergies, 254
  baby food, 254–8
  on holiday, 67
  parties, 158
  pollution, 117–18
  during pregnancy, 48–52
  safety, 50–3
Food Safety Directorate, 52–3
footwear, babies, 303
Foresight, 117, 322
formula milks, 244–6
fostering, 325–6
Foundation for the Study of Infant Deaths (FSID), 226, 320
fridges, 51–2
fruit, 255
furniture, 103, 213–17

gas and air, 143
gas detectors, 109
general anaesthetic, 145
genetic counselling, 37–8
Genetic Interest Group, 38
German measles, 54
gifts, 160–3
Gingerbread, 168, 184
glass, safety, 106–7

GP units, 18–19
GPs, 20–2
gripe waters, 204
gyms, baby, 311–12

hair, care of, 55
harnesses: car seats, 269
  highchairs, 261
  prams and buggies, 285
Health Information Service, 18
heartbeat monitors, 232
heaters, nurseries, 212
helmets, cycling, 290
herbalism, 125
highchairs, 258–60
hiring equipment, 100–2
  car seats, 270
  prams and buggies, 275
hob guards, 110
holidays: equipment, 291–4
  food, 67
  travel, 65–7, 291–6
home birth, 27
Home Office, 326
homoeopathy, 125–6
hospitals: choosing, 18–20
  consultants, 21
  disabled women, 45–6
  multiple pregnancies, 42
  National Health Service, 23–7
  private, 29–30
  suing, 326–31
  what to pack, 145–7
hygiene, food safety, 50–2
hypnosis, 127

immunization, 54
incapacity benefit, 73–4
income support, 75, 167–8
Independent Midwives Association, 28
infertility problems, 321–3
insect nets, 286
insulin, 54
insurance, travel, 66–7
interior designers, 207
International Home Birth Movement, 27
investment trusts, 81, 82, 83–4

investments, 81–5
Irish Stillbirth and Neonatal Society, 318
Irish Sudden Infant Death Society, 320
iron supplements, 49
ISSUE (National Fertility Association), 322
itchy skin, 56

John Lewis, 94

kettles, 110
kitchens, safety, 109–11

La Leche League, 235–6
labour, 137–47
　birth plans, 137–8
　father's presence, 165–6
　hypnosis, 127
　pain relief, 139–45
　problems, 326–32
　single women, 167–9
lambskin fleeces, 226
learning disabilities, parents, 46–7
Leed's Test, 34–5
Legal Aid, 330–1
legal responsibility, fathers, 164
leggings, 61–2
LIFE, 324
life-assurance savings plans, 85
lighting, nurseries, 211
listeria, 50
Littlewoods, 93
liver, in diet, 50
locking devices, prams and buggies, 286

magazines, 344
mail order, maternity clothes, 64–5
make-up, 57–8
MAMA (Meet-A-Mum Association), 333
Marks & Spencer, 95
massage, 127, 142
Maternity Alliance, 71
maternity allowance (MA), 73
maternity leave, 69–71, 148
maternity nurses, 182–3

maternity pads, 151
mats: activity, 309–10
　floor, 262
mattresses, 221–4, 320
　covers, 224
meat, 48, 50–51
medicines *see* drugs
Meet-a-Mum Association, 168–9
Meptid, 144
Metazinol, 144
microwave ovens: heating bottles in, 248–9
　sterilizers, 251
midwives: independent, 27–9
　National Health Service, 20–7
milk: cow's, 257
　expression, 240–3
　formula, 244–6
　storing breastmilk, 242–3
minerals, 119–20
mirrors, 309
miscarriage, 317–19
Miscarriage Association, 319
mobiles, 308
money *see* finances
monitors, baby, 230–2
morning sickness, 52–3
Moses baskets, 226–8, 342
Mothercare, 95–6
mother's helps, 180
mountain buggies, 280–1
muffs, 286
Multiple Births Foundation, 44
multiple births, 42–5, 282–4, 342
murals, nurseries, 210
muscles, sore, 151
music as baby gifts, 162
muslin squares, 193–4

names, choosing, 153–4
nannies, 176–80
nannyshare, 179–80
nappies, 128, 149, 187–92
nappy rash, 204
National Association of Citizens Advice Bureaux, 169
National Childbirth Trust (NCT), 20, 27, 39–41, 46, 235–6
National Childcare Campaign, 183

National Council for One-Parent Families, 169
National Foster Care Association, 326
National Health Service, 20–7, 39
National Infertility Awareness Campaign, 322
National Insurance contributions, nannies, 178
National Playbus Association, 184
National Savings, 78–80
Natural Nurturing Network, 133
nausea, 52, 54
nests, activity, 309–10
nets, prams and buggies, 286
neural-tube defects, 34, 48
New Maternity Charter, 17–18, 45
nipple cream, 239–40
nipple shields, 239
nipples, sore, 55, 151
nuchal translucency scan, 33
nurseries, childcare, 173–4
nursery: cots and cotbeds, 218–26
  decorating, 207–13
  furniture, 213–17
  monitors, 230–2
  Moses baskets, 226–8
nurses, maternity, 182–3
nursing bras, 61–2
nursing chairs, 213

one-parent benefit, 75
organic food, 118–20
osteopathy, cranial, 124–5
outdoor wear, babies, 302
oven guards, 110–11
overdrafts, 81
ovulation tests, 321–2

pagers, 101–2
pain relief: for babies, 204
  birth plans, 138
  drugs used in pregnancy, 53–4
  during labour, 139–45
paints, 208–9, 221
Parent Network, 167
Parent to Parent, 326
Parents of Prems, 150

Parent Information Network and Support (POPPINS), 150
ParentAbility, 46–7
parties, 156–9
passports, 291–2
pelican bibs, 252
pensions, state, 76
personal equity plans (PEPs), 82, 84
Pethidine, 143
photograph frames, 161
pictures, 309
piles, 55
pillows, V-shaped, for feeding, 253
Pippin Groups, 167
placenta, eating, 333–5
playgroups, 175
playpens, 103, 313–14
playsocks, 311
playtime, 305–14
PMS Help, 333
pollution, 117–18, 128
postnatal depression, 332–4
Postnatal Distress Association of Ireland, 333
prams, 274–9
Pre-School Learning Alliance, 183, 184
pregnancy: antenatal classes, 38–42, 165
  beauty care, 54–8
  benefits, 72–6
  bras, 59–61
  checklist, 337–40
  clothes, 61–5
  diet, 48–53
  disabled women, 45–7
  financial planning, 76–86
  genetic counselling, 37–8
  healthcare, 17–47
  medicines, 53–4
  miscarriage and stillbirth, 317–19
  morning sickness, 52
  multiple pregnancy, 42–5
  pregnancy tests, 323–5
  relationship problems, 317
  termination for abnormality, 319–20
  tests and screening, 30–7
  travel, 66–7
  work, 68–71

Pregnancy Advisory Service, 324
premature babies, 147–50
premium bonds, 79–80
prescriptions, free, 75–6
private health schemes, 29–30
private medicine, 30
problems, 317–36
processed foods, 51
pumps, breast, 241–2
pushchairs, 102–3, 279–87

RADAR, 47
rain covers, prams and buggies, 285
rattles, 310–11
reflexology, 127
refuges, 317
registering birth, 152–3
relationship problems, 317
restaurants, breastfeeding in, 237
rocking horses, 306
rubella, 54

safety: activity mats, 309–10
  animals, 114–16
  car travel, 266–9
  cot mattresses, 221–2
  cycling, 287–90
  in the home, 105–13
  at work, 68–9
Safeway, 96
Sainsbury, 97
salmonella, 50
SANDS (Stillbirth and Neonatal Death Society), 318–19
sanitary pads, 151
SATFA (Support Around Termination For Abnormality), 319–20
savings accounts, 77–80
scratch mitts, 301
screening, 33–7
second hand: car seats, 270
  prams and buggies, 287
sedatives, for travelling, 293–4
shared care, 22
sheep, safety, 115
sheepskin fleeces, 226
sheets, 286–7
shopping, 89–100

shopping trays, 286
sickness, 52, 54
silver gifts, 162–3
single parenthood, 167–9
skin care, 54–6
sleep bras, 61
sleep problems, 335–6
sleepsuits, 300–1
slings, 264–6
smoke detectors, 108–9
smoking, 54, 119
snowsuits, 302
soap, 201
Social Fund, 74
socks, 303
soft toys, 307
solids, introducing, 257
soothers, 228–9
sore nipples, 55
special-care baby units (SCBU), 147–8
spina bifida, 34–5
spinal block, 145
'splat' mats, 262
sponges, 201
spots, 57
sprung mattresses, 223
stair gates, 107–8
stationery, 157–8
statutory maternity pay (SMP), 72–3
steam sterilizers, 251, 293
stencils, 209
sterilizers, 251–2, 293
stickers, decorating nurseries, 209
stillbirth, 317–19
storage, toys, 215–16
stretch marks, 58
stretchsuits, 300–1
Sudden Infant Death Syndrome (SIDS), 221, 320
suing hospitals, 326–31
sunshades, prams and buggies, 285
support tights, 64
swimming: aquanatal classes, 42
  nappies for, 192
  swimwear, 64

table decorations, 158
talcum powder, 201

Index

TAMBA (Twins and Multiple Births Association), 42–3
tandem buggies, 282–3
tax, 85–6
  tax and nannies, 178
Tax-Exempt Special Savings Accounts (TESSAs), 80
teats, 246–7
teething gel, 202
TENS (transcutaneous electrical nerve stimulation), 142
termination for abnormality, 319–20
terry-towel nappies, 190–92
Tesco, 98
tests, 30–7
thermometers, 203
  bath, 200
thread veins, 56–7
three-in-one prams, 278–9
thrush, 55, 228
tights, 64, 303
toiletries:
  green, 128–30
  for postnatal mothers, 150–1
  for babies, 201–2
toothbrushes, 202
toothpaste, 202
Toxocara canis, 114–15
Toxoplasmosis, 51, 115
toys, 305–13
  environmentally friendly, 131–2
  safety, 113
  storage, 215–16
  toy libraries, 307
transport, 265–90
travel, 65–7, 291–6

travel cots, 292–3, 313–14
travel insurance, 66–7
Triple Test, 34–5
triplets, buggies, 283–4
tummy upsets, 53
twins, 42–5, 282–4, 342
two-in-one prams, 277–8

ultrasound scans, 32
umbrella-fold buggies, 281
underwear, 64
unit trusts, 81–2, 83

vaccination, 54
Vaginal Birth After Caesarean (VBAC), 21
varicose veins, 64
vegetables, 48, 255
vests, 301
vitamins, 119–20, 334
Waitrose, 99
wardrobes, 214–15
washing, baby clothes, 303–4
washing powders, 304
water birth, 140–1
weaning, 253–5, 257–8
wills, 76–7
windows, safety, 112
Women's Environmental Network, 132–3
Women's Health, 323
women's refuges, 317
Woolworth, 98
work, 68–71
Working Mother's Association, 169

zinc, 334